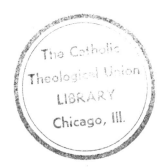

THE PATIENT AS PARTNER

Medical Ethics Series

DAVID H. SMITH AND ROBERT M. VEATCH, EDITORS

THE
PATIENT
AS
PARTNER

A Theory of
Human-Experimentation Ethics

Robert M. Veatch

Indiana
University
Press

BLOOMINGTON AND INDIANAPOLIS

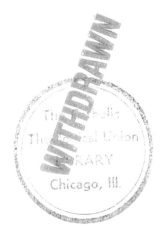

Manufactured in the United States of America

Library of Congress Cataloging-in-Publication Data

Veatch, Robert M.
The patient as partner.

(Medical ethics series)
Most of the essays included are edited and revised
versions of essays originally written from 1971–1983.
1. Human experimentation in medicine—Moral and
ethical aspects. 2. Patient compliance. 3. Medical
ethics. I. Title. II. Series. [DNLM: 1. Ethics,
Medical—essays. 2. Human Experimentation—essays.
3. Patient Advocacy—essays. 4. Professional-Patient
Relations—essays. W 50 V395p]
R853.H8V43 1987 174'.28 86-45043
ISBN 0-253-35725-X

2 3 4 5 91 90 89

To Regina B. Veatch
and Cecil R. Veatch

CONTENTS

PART V. Special Research Contexts

PART VI. Emerging Themes and Controversies

PREFACE

The past twenty years has been a time of turbulence for medical ethics. What once was essentially a professional domain dominated by pious references to Hippocrates has become the concern of thinking laypeople worried about decisions being made in medicine. The recognition that new biomedical technology and new medical research really have important impacts—for better or worse—on human lives is part of the reason. The egalitarian rights revolution of the 1960s aroused in all of us a concern for the relatively powerless: in civil rights, women's and students' rights, and, inevitably, the rights of patients. These two forces—the advances in biomedical technology and the rising consciousness of the rights of the weaker parties of relationships—generated what can, without exaggeration, be called a revolution in medical ethics. A new medical ethics has emerged within this period, one that is much less exclusively concerned about the traditional Hippocratic agenda of having clinicians do what they think will benefit patients (even if patients do not concur) and much more concerned about protecting the rights of patients as well as the broader social, ethical questions of resource allocation and justice.

This new, broader medical ethic is influenced by traditions largely outside of medicine. The Hippocratic tradition has been less concerned about affirming the dignity of the individual and protecting the most needy in the community than the Judeo-Christian tradition has been. That tradition has certainly fed the new medical ethic that has emerged. At least as important has been the secular tradition of liberal political philosophy. It is here that the principle of autonomy as well as justice has emerged full-blown as a new foundation for medical ethics.

In *A Theory of Medical Ethics* I attempted to construct a general theoretical formulation of this new ethic in which laypeople as well as professionals were seen as active, full participants in medical decisions. It was clear that in that volume I could only sketch the broadest outlines of the covenant or contract medical ethic with its emphasis on laypersons as key actors in medical decisions. At the time it was clear that this approach had implications for many spheres of medicine and many specific problems within medicine that would need to be developed much more fully. One such area for further development was the lay-professional relationship in research and clinical medicine. I postponed for another time the enormous project of developing these implications. The time has come to start making good on that project.

In April of 1982 I was asked to deliver the David Barap Brin Lecture of Ethical Issues in Clinical Cancer Research at the Johns Hopkins Oncology Center. It was an occasion devoted to remembering one of the Center's patients, a bright, articulate twenty-three-year-old dying of leukemia, who had an unusual impact on the Center staff. I did not have the privilege of knowing this remarkable young man, yet the picture I get is one of a warm, intelligent, serious human being who recognized that he had a role to play in the structuring of his clinical care. One of the medical staff involved in caring for David Brin described him to me as "an inquisitive, thoughtful young man who was loved by those who participated in his care." My impression was one of a patient who recognized that his own life had something to contribute to the decisions about his care and, as it turns out, to the care of others at Johns Hopkins.

It was during the preparation of that lecture that the concept of the patient as an active partner in the design and execution of medical research came to me as a symbol of the new image of the layperson in the new medical ethics. It is testimony to the clinicians at Johns Hopkins that they recognized the importance of this symbol and, rather than rebelling against it, encouraged further explorations into the relationship between researcher/clinicians and this new breed of patients who were more than objects to be manipulated for the good of science. My *Theory of Medical Ethics* had appeared not long before I wrote the lecture, and I had been thinking of ways that the implications of the overall theory could be made clear for more specific medical areas such as human-subjects research. I chose the "patient as partner" theme for that lecture as a way of gathering my thoughts and writing on this subject. Drawing on what turned out to be a rather extensive collection of essays on specific issues of human-subjects research, I traced the implications of a patient-centered contract or covenant ethic for experimentation with human subjects.

The present volume is the result. The previously published essays were originally written over the period from 1971 to 1983; they reflect evolution in the debate over medical ethics, my own thoughts on the subject, the federal regulations, and state law. I have edited and, where necessary, added to the essays in order to produce a systematic discussion.

Three of the chapters have not appeared in any published form previously. I had written essays on autonomy and justice as basic principles, but had never actually developed an essay on the principle of beneficence as it relates to human experimentation. That essay was prepared especially for this volume and appears as chapter 2.

A central theme of this volume is that if the patient is an active partner in the relationship, then he or she must be adequately informed not only about the risks and benefits of the research, but also of the purposes, methods, alternatives, and so forth. Moreover, since reasonable researchers (as well as reasonable medical ethicists) may differ from reasonable potential subjects on the question of what they would want to know about research before deciding whether to participate, the most obvious way to satisfy the reasonable-person criterion whenever there is any doubt is to go ask a group of potential subjects, hence the idea of using surrogate-subject panels. I had the opportunity to work on this idea with Richard Winer, now a physician practicing in Smyrna, Georgia, during his internship at the Hastings Center in New York. In collaboration with Victor Sidel, Chairman of the Department of Social Medicine at Montefiore Hospital and Chairman of Montefiore's institutional review board, and Morton Spivack, of the Departments of Medicine and Pathology at Montefiore Hospital and Albert Einstein College of Medicine, we had the opportunity to test out the model of surrogate-subject panels. That study, which illustrates the implications of the patient-as-partner methodology, has never been published previously. I am grateful to my co-authors for permission to include it in this volume. The third chapter that has never been published previously is the final chapter, the summing up of emerging themes of controversies.

The remaining chapters have been edited to varying degrees. In all cases I have attempted to bring the references, especially the references to federal regulations, up to date. A great number of people have helped me over the years in developing my thinking about a theory of the ethics of human experimentation that would involve the patient or subject as an active, full participant in the research process. I have served on three different institutional review boards (IRBs). First, I served briefly as chairman of a small committee at the Institute of Society, Ethics and the Life Sciences that was responsible for reviewing research, primarily social-science and interview research, conducted at the Institute. From 1975–1980 I was privileged to be a member of the IRB at Montefiore Hospital in the Bronx. Then from 1980 until the present I have served as a member of the IRB for the National Institute of Occupational Health and Safety (NIOSH). To Victor Sidel, the chairman at Montefiore; to Ralph Yodaiken and Barry Johnson, the chairmen of the NIOSH board; and to the members of all three boards, I am particularly grateful. The long hours of argument over hundreds of research protocols have been an education. Over those years I have grown to respect the care and dedication with which these IRB members approach their task. I have learned new perspectives, new arguments, and new sensitivities from each.

I wish to express special appreciation to John Fetting, M.D., at Johns Hopkins for first inviting me to give the Brin Lecture and for encouraging comments about the manuscript, and I thank the Brin family for making that lecture possible. I am also grateful to Marcia Sichol, Kathleen Buckley, Maura O'Brien, Caren Kieswetter, and particularly to Donna Horak Mitsock, who helped in editing, revising, and updating every chapter of the volume.

It is only an accident that the first area of application of this new patient-centered contract or covenant theory of medical ethics is human experimentation. The same thesis, that the patient should be seen as an active partner participating in medical decisions as a key or central actor by bringing his or her own system of beliefs and values to these decisions, is equally relevant to routine clinical medicine. A second volume dealing with the therapeutic relation between layperson and professional will be needed to complete the project. That, however, will have to wait until another day.

ACKNOWLEDGMENTS

Chapter 1 was adapted from an article that first appeared as "The Patient as Partner: Ethics in Clinical Oncology Research," *Johns Hopkins Medical Journal* 151 (October 1982):155–61; and "Human Experimentation—Ethical Questions Persist," *Hastings Center Report* 3 (No. 3, June 1973):1–3.

Chapter 2 is an original article prepared for this volume.

Chapter 3 is based in part on "Three Theories of Informed Consent: Philosophical Foundations and Policy Implications," *The Belmont Report: Ethical Principles and Guidelines for the Protection of Human Subjects of Research* (Washington, D.C.: National Commission for the Protection of Human Subjects of Biomedical and Behavioral Research, DHEW Publication No. (05)78–0014), pp. 26–1 through 26–66.

Chapters 4 and 9 are adapted from "Justice and Research Design: The Case for a Semi-Randomization Clinical Trial," *Clinical Research* 31 (February 1983):12–22.

Chapter 5 is adapted from "Federal Regulation of Medicine and Biomedical Research: Power, Authority, and Legitimacy," in *The Law-Medicine Relation: A Philosophical Exploration*, ed. S. F. Spicker, J. M. Healey, and H. T. Englehardt, Jr. (Dordrecht, Holland: D. Reidel Publishing Co., 1981), pp. 75–91.

Chapter 6 is based in part on "The National Commission Recommendations on IRBs," *Hastings Center Report* 9 (No. 1, February 1979):22–28; and on "Protecting Human Subjects: The Federal Government Steps Back," *Hastings Center Report* 11 (June 1981):9–12; as well as on previously unpublished material.

Chapter 7 first appeared in a somewhat different form as "Human Experimentation Committees: Professional or Representative?" *Hastings Center Report* 5 (October 1975):31–40.

Chapter 8 first appeared in a somewhat different form as "Liability and the IRB Member: The Ethical Aspects," *IRB* 1 (No. 3, May 1979):8–9.

Chapter 10 is adapted from "Human Experimentation: The Crucial Choices Ahead," *Prism* 2 (No. 7, July 1974):58–61, 71. Used by permission of the American Medical Association.

Chapter 11 first appeared as "Longitudinal Studies, Sequential Design, and Grant Renewals: What to Do with Preliminary Data," *IRB* 1 (No. 4, June/July 1979):1–3.

Chapter 12 has not previously been published. I am grateful to Drs. Winer, Sidel, and Spivack for permission to include it in this volume.

Chapter 13 is adapted from "Limits to the Right of Privacy: Reason, Not Rhetoric," *IRB* 4 (April 1982):5–7.

Chapter 14 first appeared as "Experimental Pregnancy: The Ethical Complexities of Experimentation with Oral Contraceptives," *Hastings Center Report* 1 (June 1971):2–3.

Chapter 15 is based on "Beyond Consent to Treatment," *IRB* 3 (February 1981):7–8.

Chapter 16 is adapted from "Research on 'Non-consentables'," *IRB* 3 (January 1981):6–7.

Chapter 17 first appeared in somewhat different form as "Case Study: Risk-Taking in Cancer Chemotherapy," *IRB* 1 (No. 5, August/September 1979):4–6.

Chapter 18 first appeared as "The Ethics of Research Involving Radiation," *IRB* 4 (January 1982):3–5.

Chapter 19 was prepared for this volume.

PART

I

Introduction

CHAPTER ONE

The Patient as Partner

In 1966 Henry Beecher first published his *New England Journal of Medicine* exposé describing blatantly unethical research methodologies.[1] We have made enormous strides since the days when we would purposely leave syphilis untreated in a group of poor, black southern men in order to study the course of untreated disease.[2] We no longer see research protocols where Mexican-American women are given placebos in place of birth-control pills to learn more about the psychogenic origins of reported side effects of the pill.[3] We look back appalled at the thought that researchers would inject live cancer cells into terminally ill patients without their knowledge in order to test a hypothesis about the body's rejection mechanisms.[4]

These ethical outrages of an earlier era have forced us as a community to reassess the ethics of clinical research and to formulate a set of moral and legal guidelines providing a mandate for ethically acceptable research. We now have a literature on informed consent, on the principles of confidentiality, and on the trading off of risks to subjects for the potential benefits to mankind. We live in the post-Nuremberg era.

Now we have gone about as far as we can go in trying to clarify the ethics of clinical research by debating specific topics in the context of an isolated example of some ethical outrage. In fact, we must be even more critical than that.

The ethical abuses that have formed the background of much of our problem-oriented medical ethical reflection represented rather rare aberrations even in their own era. The serious problems that command the newspaper headlines and the attention of senators investigating the clinical-research enterprise constitute a deviant pattern in medical research. Most researchers, even in the 1940s and 50s, were not misanthropes—mad scientists bent on producing their results at the expense of unknowing victim-subjects. Rather, they were as they are today—dedicated, concerned human beings struggling with difficult clinical and ethical problems.

We may well have been misled into thinking that the medical ethics of clinical research can be settled by generating a few simple moral rules based on rather ad hoc reflections and common sense. However, the time for easy ethics is over; what is needed is a new way of getting at the real clinical ethical problems facing the community of researchers and patients in the clinical research centers of this country and the rest of the world. We need some framework for dealing with the real-life ethical problems, not the more obvious ethical abuses.

We do not need an ethic that will tell us that patients should be told of obvious, serious risks of side effects from a multi-drug chemotherapeutic trial; we know that. We need some mechanism for deciding just how many of the countless smaller risks and concerns of the researcher should be discussed with the patient. We do not need an ethic that will tell us that it is immoral to continue to give a placebo after a drug has been shown beyond doubt to be effective. We need an ethic that will deal with the stickier problem of when to stop a protocol prematurely, as was done not long ago with the propranolol study for myocardial infarction.[5] We need an ethic that will tell us whether we should discuss with patients preliminary trends in the data even if it compromises the research protocol. We do not need an ethic that tells us it is immoral to provide toxic levels of whole-body radiation without adequate consent;[6] we need one that tells us whether we should ask patients receiving methotrexate with leucovorin rescue to follow the slightly riskier course of taking their leucovorin at home in order to save money for the clinical center.[7] We do not need to be told it is unethical to force recent kidney transplant recipients to stand to the point of fainting immediately after transplant surgery. We need an ethic that will say something about how many extra IV taps are acceptable in a patient who is already so filled with needle marks that he cannot stand the sight of another syringe or how many extra trips to the clinic should be imposed on patients whose lives have been reduced to an endless series of stretcher transports.

We need to get at the real ethical issues of medical research, not just the ad hoc list of rules that eliminate the more obvious abuses. In order to do that, we are going to have to get behind the more problem-oriented codes and rules and regulations to understand what the real ethical foundations of the ethics of research ought to be so that research subjects can be treated as respected, dignified, moral agents.

In the past, research subjects have all too often been treated as passive "material" suitable for providing additional data points. This stems in part from the presumption that clinical research subjects are sick, usually very sick, and thus not capable of autonomous decision-making or full, active participation in the research. In fact, the true nature of research subjects is much more complex. Many are "normals" participating in phase I clinical trials to determine safety of drugs or serving as controls in studies in which they themselves are in no way debilitated. Others are suffering from chronic disease that in no way jeopardizes their capacity to think, feel, reason, and express judgments about their participation as well as broader questions about the design and purposes of the research. Still others—those relatively rare subjects who are suffering from acute illness that leaves them incapacitated to some extent—have developed life-style patterns, beliefs, and values that can be determined and incorporated into judgments about their participation. Finally, even in cases where the subject is not competent to participate actively in the research—in cases of infants, the mentally disabled, and the senile, for example—someone else is normally in the guardian role. That person can take on the role of active agent cooperating with the investigator-team in critical decisions that affect the subject as well as the research. In all cases, either the subjects themselves or their agents can be active, moral agents. They should be treated as human beings with dignity and respect.

This picture of the lay decision-maker as a questioning, thinking, feeling, active moral person may give us some insight into the foundation of an ethic for research. It is a picture radically different from two other pictures that one sometimes gets of the way subjects for medical research are thought of by researchers.

It is radically different from viewing the subject as "research material," as a useful substance necessary to complete the research objectives. The image of the subject as "research material" is suggested by some older protocols such as the studies when cortisone was first used for patients suffering from arthritis. After dramatic results were obtained from the initial cortisone trials, the subjects were switched over to a placebo in order to demonstrate that their arthritic pain would return when the cortisone administration was stopped. The researchers demonstrated that the pain did indeed return and, upon completion of the study, sent their subjects home. There seemed to be no grasping of the fact that these were real-life, flesh-and-blood, suffering human beings who had been used for research and then sent away to return to their misery. If we begin thinking of subjects as active, autonomous agents participating in the research along with the researcher, the idea of the subject as "research material" will disappear forever.

The idea of an inquisitive, active, moral human being also rules out the image of a research subject as a patient—in the negative sense that word originally implied—as one who is passively ministered unto—as one who because of his or her illness loses all the capacity to think, feel, reason, and participate actively in medical decision making along with the researchers. The old Hippocratic ethic saw the patient as a weak, debilitated, childlike victim, incapable of functioning as a real moral agent.

Instead, we need to think of the subject as neither research material nor passive patient, but simply as a *person*, with all the moral overtones that that word conveys. As such, it is appropriate to view the person as a *partner* in the research enterprise. The result is a radically different and new moral basis for the relationship between the researcher and the research subject.

Now, of course, not all those who are candidates for participation in human-subjects research can be thought of as partners. Some will be suffering from an acute illness where instantaneous decisions must be made. Others will be so debilitated by their illness that they themselves cannot actively participate at the moment of critical decision making. Still others may be too young, too old, or too out of communication with reality to play this role as partner in the research. Even in those cases, however, they may participate indirectly. They may participate through wishes they have expressed and through a life-style they have developed in their healthier moments; they may participate through their families. Often the family as a unit bears the burden of participation in research and the responsibility for protecting the rights and welfare of their sick members.

Patients with chronic disease such as cancer are an ideal example of persons who can be viewed as partners in the research enterprise. The disease course is often prolonged, giving patients as well as families an extended period to learn about the illness and to understand the current state of medical problems in treating it. The illness often goes through cycles of remission and relapse so that, at least at times, persons who are ill may feel quite comfortable discussing their condition and the treatment options, including the experimental ones. In short, research on chronic illness is an ideal setting for experimenting not only with new treatment regimens, but also with new models for researcher/subject relationships including relationships where the subject is viewed as an active partner in the common struggle.

The researcher/subject relationship is intriguing, especially as it differs from the more traditional physician/patient relationship. There is often a mutual dependence that is missing in the more traditional therapeutic relationship, making the metaphor of partners particularly appropriate. In the traditional therapeutic relationship, the patient is often seen as having enormous need for the physician, but, by contrast, the physician cannot really be said to *need* his or her patients. Of course, the good physician has made a commitment to benefit patients or to serve them, and he or she cannot fulfill that commitment unless patients are available. Of course, professionals need clients economically in order to survive to practice their profession. But the researcher needs subjects in quite a different way. Clinical researchers simply cannot complete their life mission unless subjects are willing to step forward and help them. At times, researchers are almost placed in a position of begging for help from potential subjects (whether or not they admit to subjects that is what they are doing). It is a relationship not dissimilar to the desperate need sick laypersons feel for someone with professional medical skills that may help them. The two are really mutually dependent in a way that is both moving and hopeful. There is a real possibility for a kind of active collaboration that today exists only rarely between professionals and laypeople.

This is not to suggest that this relationship has the makings of one in which the researcher and the subject need to become close friends—become pals. That may happen, but normally it will not. It is not necessary that it should, perhaps better if it does not. The metaphor of partners is exact. Partners normally come together not because they share exactly the same interests and abilities, but because there is some mutuality of interests, some common point of intersection where each can help the other. Business partnerships and marriages often work best if the partners possess complementary skills and aptitudes.

It should be very clear that the patient as partner in the research enterprise will have an agenda that differs from that of the researcher. For researchers, it is often only honest to admit that their primary interest is in learning about a disease and its treatment for the benefit of future patients. Of course, in a real and dedicated way they will be concerned about the welfare of the present patient—at least if that researcher views the subject as a partner. By contrast, research subjects will have as their primary interest their own immediate medical needs and the welfare of those with whom they are close. They, in turn, may have some real interest in the more general, vague, abstract benefits to others that may eventually accrue—especially if they have developed an identification with their fellow sufferers. But the two agendas are different; they overlap—that is what makes a partnership possible—but they are different.

Since patients as partners have agendas of their own, they may very well bring to the research preferences, values, ethics, and belief systems that differ from those of researchers. It may be rational for the subject to choose one course of action when, from the researcher's point of view, there is no medical basis for choosing one course rather than another.

Consider an ongoing chemotherapy protocol designed to treat adolescents with leukemia. Originally, the standard treatment with the agent in question had been five years—five years of intermittent nausea, alopecia, and other rather traumatic effects on the young patients. The regimen had been lowered to three years with no statistically significant decline in mortality, and everyone was thrilled. The researchers were now considering an experiment where patients would be randomized into two arms: One group would receive the agent for three years (the now-standard treatment), and the other (the experimental arm) would receive it for two years. They were concerned about a possible slight increase in mortality although they had good reason to believe that the increase, if there was any, would be very small. On the other hand, if they could lower the treatment time to two years, the youngsters would be spared one year's worth of unpleasant and psychologically traumatic side effects.

The researchers made every effort to explain to the patients and their parents the potential advantages and disadvantages of each treatment arm. They said that in their judgment there was no clear reason to choose one arm rather than the other (a standard requirement if randomized clinical trials are to be considered ethical). After the randomization process was complete, one girl and her mother were told that the girl had been placed in the three-year arm of the study. At that point, the researchers were not prepared for the girl's response and that of her mother. They both broke down in tears.

Intervention from the social worker and several conversations with the researchers led to some clarification. The girl and her mother had hoped desperately that she would be placed in the two-year arm. What in the world was happening? Did the girl and her mother realize that they had a chance to get the two-year treatment regimen by refusing to be in the study and taking the readily available compound as part of standard therapy, stopping after two years instead of the normal three years? Were they behaving irrationally (since there was no clear medical evidence one way or the other that one arm would be better than the other)? Were there some deeper psychological factors that no one involved was able to understand—for example, did the girl and her mother perceive the randomization as a lack of caring on the part of the clinicians? Did their being placed in a study convey (falsely, in this case) that their situation was particularly hopeless? We simply do not know what was going on.

It is clear that research subjects may rationally prefer one treatment arm of a randomized clinical trial (RCT) rather than another even if there is no medical reason for the choice. They might have been saying in this case that the agony of the side effects was so great to the girl that, for them, the expected slight increased mortality risk would have been well worth it if they could have gotten into the two-year arm. While two options in a clinical trial are the same medically, they will amost always differ psychologically, physically, or socially for the subject. Only in the rarest of circumstances will active subjects really be indifferent to the two treatment options if indeed they really understand what these options are. That they choose to participate at all under these circumstances is testimony to the partnership that is created. Of course they may have to participate in some cases in order to get any chance of getting an experimental treatment. In many other cases, they do so out of a real desire to see progress made in treating their condition (even if they themselves do not benefit). Sometimes it is a pure sense of altruism that moves the subject, like that girl and her mother, to say "yes" to the request to participate.

What we are left with is a convergence of interests where both researcher and subject have something to gain by participating and where each is called upon to make some sacrifice for the benefit of the other. These are the true makings of a partnership, if only it is allowed to flourish. It is also the potential foundation for an ethics of research, especially in a chronic-disease research setting such as a clinical cancer research center. It is an ethical foundation that is radically different from either of the two traditional ethics for clinical research: the utilitarian ethic where the goal is to produce the greatest good for the greatest number even if it means using the subject as a means to an end and the Hippocratic ethic where the goal is to benefit the patient even as the patient remains a passive, uninvolved recipient of the researcher's kindness. If researcher and subject are seen as partners who are both autonomous, responsible, dignified human agents coming together to form a limited covenant for pursuit of mutual interest, virtually all aspects of the ethics of clinical research are affected. It provides a new foundation for ethically acceptable clinical research.

THE IMPLICATIONS FOR THREE SPECIFIC PROBLEMS

The idea of the patient as partner—the notion of a social covenant binding researcher and subject—will affect several of the most timely, most novel, most controversial issues in clinical research. What does this new foundation mean for the reasonable-person doctrine in informed consent, the handling of preliminary data, and the designing of research with the idea that the subject is a partner?

THE REASONABLE PERSON DOCTRINE IN INFORMED CONSENT

Informed consent is by now one of the oldest, most obvious requirements of ethically acceptable research. We have lists of the appropriate elements for disclosure, rules for obtaining and documenting the consent, and review boards that verify the process.[8] What is not realized is that different ethical foundations for the consent requirement lead, in some cases, to very different moves in discussing the proposed research with the subject. Under the Hippocratic ethic where the researcher's first mission is to benefit the patient and protect his or her welfare, the information transmitted in a consent process is designed to make sure the patient's interests are protected. Subjects are told of the risks, potential side effects, and available, alternative treatments. In rare cases, however, it is believed that certain pieces of information might harm the subjects—might upset them psychologically or even cause so much distress that they would irrationally withdraw from the study. If the old Hippocratic, patient-benefit ethic underlies the consent process, it is not only permissible, but is actually required that such disturbing elements of information be omitted from the consent process. We used to call this the therapeutic privilege, the old paternalism in its rawest form.

If the foundation of the consent process is the utilitarian ethic of producing the greatest good for the greatest number, then the consent process is even more tenuous. One gets consent whenever it furthers the research—when it is necessary to recruit subjects or protect the reputation of the institution—but not simply because the subject has a right to it. It is an ethic that would justify the Nazi experiments if only the Nazis had been clever enough to design really beneficial research. In extreme cases where good for society could be done only by omitting consent, the omission is easily justified.

The idea of the patient as partner provides a totally new reason for informing the potential subject of the research. It is not at all because it would benefit the patient or benefit the society, but simply because it is impossible for one to participate in the research enterprise as a full partner—as a substantially autonomous, respected, dignified human being—without knowing what is going on.

The idea of the patient as partner also gives us a new basis for determining how much information to transmit to the potential subject. Some zealots for informed consent sometimes talk about "full consent" or "complete information," but no one ever gets fully informed consent. It is literally impossible to transmit it all. No one in his right mind would even want to know all that the researcher knows. It would involve too much time, too much trivia.

What is to be transmitted then? The patient as a partner needs to know all those things that a reasonable person would want to know in order to decide whether to participate in the partnership.[9] Reasonable persons who are potential partners in a venture may want to know certain risks and potential benefits, but they may also want to know information that has no bearing whatsoever on potential risks. They may want to know something about the purpose of the study, maybe even something about the theory underlying the innovation. It is no longer a matter of benefits and harms—to either the subject or the society—but rather what it takes to decide whether to become an active partner in an important enterprise.

The question of how much information to transmit then becomes an empirical one. In principle, it cannot be answered, or answered well, by researchers, philosophers, lawyers, or IRB members sitting around speculating on what people would like to know. Anyone with special expertise in research or philosophy or law or the regulatory process may have a very unique set of desires about how much information people would want to know. The only way to determine accurately what reasonable subjects would want to know is to ask them. Experiments are actually under way sampling groups drawn from the same populations as research subjects asking them, for example, whether they would want to be told that blood donated to a blood bank might be used for research rather than for therapeutic purposes. They have been asked in fascinating research by Ruth Faden how many of the side effects of Dilantin they would like to be told about.[10]

Recent debate over the use of the reasonable-person standard has led to a new controversy about what should happen when the individual subject differs in some way from the typical reasonable person. Must the researcher disclose what the subject would want to know or what the typical reasonable person would want to know? If the model is one of the subject participating as an active partner, the answer becomes clear. The goal is to provide whatever information is needed for the subject to make an informed choice about participating, that is, what this particular subject would want to know.

This creates a potentially serious problem. It is hard enough for the researcher to determine what the typical reasonable person would want to know. It seems like an impossible burden to expect researchers to determine each idiosyncratic special concern of each unique subject. If the typical reasonable person were used as the standard for deciding what information to transmit, obviously mistakes would be made at the margin. If the subjects are to participate as *active* partners, they are going to bear some responsibility at this point. The researcher will have to disclose those things about the study that a typical reasonable person would want to know, but the potential subject will have the obligation to signal if he or she wants more or less information or specialized information of some sort. That is appropriate if the subject is an active, full participant in the process. The researcher's job will be to create a climate where the subject can express uniqueness in this way.

PRELIMINARY DATA

The model of the patient as partner also sheds light on a second, even more difficult, controversial new area of debate in research ethics. It is increasingly becoming apparent that trends emerge in data at a point prior to the time when an adequate level of significance is reached. In multi-center studies, such as those of the Eastern Cooperative Oncology Group, neither researchers nor subjects may be aware of patterns as they emerge. The question now being raised is whether subjects should be told anything about those preliminary trends.

Obviously, the orthodox view is that it is bad science to disclose data prematurely. It might taint the findings if later subjects in a study are given different information than earlier subjects. More than that, it might well lead to a decision by later subjects to withdraw from the study in order to obtain the treatment that is showing up more favorably in the early returns.

Consider the example of the adolescent girl and her mother randomized between two and three years of chemotherapy for leukemia. Suppose the design were sequential and the present pattern was one in which the mortality rate of the two-year treatment arm was five percent higher than the mortality rate of the three-year arm among those who had entered the protocol at least five years previously, but that the difference was statistically significantly different only at the $p = 0.1$ level. From the point of good science, it seems clear that the study should continue until a more attractive significance level is reached (such as $p = 0.05$). Some might be tempted to say that it would be irrational for someone to choose the three-year arm rather than the two-year arm at this point (since the significance level is not yet low enough). That is correct from the point of view of the scientists. They should not yet publish results claiming that the three-year arm is better than the two-year arm. From the patient's point of view, however, there is no opportunity to wait until more data are in. She (and her mother) must choose to enter the study or to refuse. If they refuse, they can take their original choice of the two-year arm—which they preferred for socially important reasons—or they can now choose the three-year treatment. They would be doing so on shaky data, but if the null hypothesis is rejected at the 0.1 level, they have a much better than fifty-fifty chance of being correct in acting on the assumption that there is a difference. Clearly, choosing three years would be the rational thing to do from a clinical perspective of a patient forced to one treatment option or the other who now desired to make death prevention the definitive criterion.

The result of all this is a terrible mess for clinical research. If we ask whether the reasonable person would want to know of a preliminary data trend, the answer is almost certain to be positive, especially for major therapeutic choices such as the life-and-death choices in research. If the research dealt with a relatively minor therapeutic objective—relieving minor headache, for example—rational patients might be willing to forego this knowledge in order to advance science. Some subjects might be willing to even in oncology, but it would be asking a great deal of the subject.

The three alternative foundations for an ethic of research provide very different answers to this problem. If the subject is viewed as "research material" in the traditional utilitarian ethic of the greatest good for the greatest number, there is, of course, no reason to tell the subject at all—unless word of the non-disclosure gets out and harms the institution's reputation. If the ethic is the old Hippocratic, patient-benefitting ethic, it seems the subject must be told of even very preliminary trends. In fact, virtually all research medicine is morally unacceptable to a physician working strictly in the Hippocratic tradition because in research, by its very nature, the physician is working not simply to benefit the patient, but primarily to benefit others.

The model of the patient as partner provides an interesting compromise. Certainly the subject/partner must be told those things that a reasonable person would want to know. In this model they are, after all, autonomous, dignified participants in the study. However, there remain two possible ways out of this dilemma. First, reasonable subjects may agree that certain very preliminary trends might be withheld from them—on the grounds that they consent to being altruistic at least to this extent. Second, even if reasonable persons would want to know about the preliminary data, they may still, if they view themselves as full partners in an important research enterprise, be willing to agree to remain blind as to which group they are in, thus permitting the research to go to completion. Of course, if the data trend is substantial (fifty percent less death at the $p = 0.06$ level), the rational subject may have to forego the opportunity to be a partner in the project, and the researcher will have to face the awful problem of figuring out how to complete the study.

DESIGNING RESEARCH TO BENEFIT SUBJECTS

There is a third new area of controversy in clinical research that can be clarified using the model of the patient as partner. Recent new Department of Health and Human Services (DHHS) requirements put into federal regulation what the National Commission for the Protection of Human

Subjects had recommended and philosophers have anticipated: They have insisted on equity in selection of subjects and in the design of research.[11]

Suppose there are two ways to design a piece of research. The first when compared to the second is somewhat better science but places the subjects at slightly greater risk of harm or inconvenience. The research involving methotrexate with leucovorin rescue provides a clear example. In such studies, massive "overdoses" of the chemotherapeutic agent methotrexate are given which are reversed some hours or days later with the compound leucovorin. In one case, the researchers proposed to administer the leuco-vorin by having the patients take home oral doses which they would take under their own supervision. They were operating out of the traditional research utilitarian ethic of the greatest good for the greatest number.

Two kinds of objections emerged when this protocol was reviewed by an IRB. The followers of the old Hippocratic ethic objected that the risk to the patient was too great. A patient who forgot (or purposely omitted) the leucovorin would be in substantial jeopardy, would perhaps die. Further-more, the administration of the drug and the side effects could be monitored more carefully if the patients were hospitalized at the clinical center. Hospi-talize them "in order to protect them" was their argument.

The second objection came from those who took the perspective of what might be called the patient as partner. They said neither benefit to the patient nor benefit to the society can be the decisive moral criterion. Some patients might prefer the freedom of being able to take the leucovorin at home. It would avoid several days of hospitalization in each three-week cycle of the methotrexate administration. They should have the right to do so even if it is risky and even if it is not quite as elegant scientifically. On the other hand, if some patients are concerned about the risk and desire the closer supervision—if they are not distressed by the inconvenience of hospitaliza-tion—they should have the right to hospitalization. They proposed that patients be viewed as active participants in the design of the research. They should be asked whether they would rather get the leucovorin at home or in the hospital. The researchers could offer two separate studies or, if they chose, one study with two modes of administration. The results would not be quite as elegant or efficient—it would even be riskier—but they would end up treating the subjects as autonomous, responsible partners in designing the research.

If the patient is regarded as a partner in the research, similar compro-mises in research design might be required to maintain the dignity of the patient and to assure that family and friends are available for comfort, support, and companionship when the subject wants them. Sometimes—as in the leucovorin rescue—the partnership model provides a justification for what the researcher wants to do that might otherwise be unavailable.

THE PATIENT-AS-PARTNER RESEARCH AGENDA

The patient-as-partner model as a foundation for an ethic of research should not be expected to produce any quick, definitive answers for the difficult ethical questions that have been raised. The problems of what constitutes informed consent, whether to apprise subjects of preliminary data, and how to insure humane and equitable design of research are all difficult, complex issues. It would be expecting miracles to believe that the development of a new ethical concept could immediately solve all of them.

Instead, it provides a new framework for beginning to think about these problems—a new research agenda for the ethics of medical research. Dr. Faden's work at Johns Hopkins on the reasonable-person standard is an example of some intriguing work already in process. Other research might be undertaken in this area as well. Will it be possible to develop mechanisms for asking groups of subjects how much information should be transmitted for consent to be reasonably informed? What should happen when some reasonable subjects want a piece of information and others do not? How reliable an approximation of the reasonable-subject standard is produced when researchers of IRBs guess at what subjects would want to be told?

The preliminary data problem generates a research agenda, too. At what point would reasonable subjects decline to participate in a randomization if they knew about a preliminary data trend? Are there identifiable sociological characteristics of those who agree to be randomized after hearing of preliminary data? Are there identifiable characteristics of those who agree to be randomized without knowing of the data trend? Does that in fact signal a bias in the sample that makes existing subject pools suspect (because only special types of people are willing to be randomized in the face of lack of knowledge about the data)?

Of all the implications of the model of the patient as partner, the most provocative for new research agendas in medical ethics may be the one generated out of concern for making the subject of research a full, active participant in the design of research. This may come in the form of developing ways to respond to the subject's need for greater comfort and convenience in the course of research. It may come in adjustments that are made to involve family and friends more responsibly and humanely. It may come in actual changes in the protocol designed to increase the benefits to the subject even if it means compromising certain other benefits of the research.

We simply have never studied the problem of how benefits to the subjects should be considered in comparison to benefits to others. We have never systematically sought the active participation of the subjects in the design of research. If subjects are viewed as active, responsible partners in the research—as partners in an important social-scientific process—then these questions will have to be addressed. The research agenda for medical ethics is rich. The idea of the patient as partner in medical research has other implications that have just begun to be explored: If subjects are active partners in the research, is there an obligation to share financial rewards? Or to share the sense of accomplishment?

It is exciting to think about the possibility of viewing the patient as partner in at least certain kinds of research. We have always known that the

patient as subject contributes an essential element to the research enterprise. Radically new potential for subject involvement is on the horizon if
only we respond sensitively to the needs and interests of the patient, making
them and their families, whenever possible, full partners in the process. The
result may well be better science; it is certain to be better ethics.

PART

II

*The Foundations of an
Ethic of Experimentation*

CHAPTER TWO

Doing Good: Beneficence as the Minimal Justification for Research

Any research on human subjects must have the potential of doing some good. That seems obvious. There may be room for disagreement over what counts as a good. Advancing knowledge per se, for instance, according to some theories of value is a good and may be sufficient to justify research. According to other notions of value, knowledge itself might not be sufficient. But some good must come of the exposure of human beings to the risks, inconveniences, and nuisance of research investigations. That is the insight derived from what is sometimes referred to as the principle of beneficence—the principle that a right-making characteristic of action is that it produces good consequences. Such a view is suggested by the remark of the nineteenth-century physiologist Claude Bernard, sometimes thought of as the father of experimental medicine, when he said that:

> Christian morals forbid only one thing, doing ill to one's neighbor. So, among the experiments that may be tried in man, those that can only do harm are forbidden, those that are innocent are permissible, and those that may do good are obligatory.[1]

BENEFICENCE AS A MINIMUM

No stronger, clearer statement of the researcher's imperative has ever been articulated. Yet surely Bernard has overstated his case. If every research idea that may do good is obligatory, then every researcher, indeed every physician, even every layperson, whenever confronted with a research idea that may do some good would have to stop whatever he or she is doing and run off

16

to do research. If Bernard were taken seriously this would apply even in cases where the good is only a possibility, even cases where harm is an even more likely possibility.

Bernard, writing in 1865 just two years after Mill published his *Utilitarianism*, has given us the purest, simplest, if most naive, application of the principle of beneficence to research medicine. The principle of beneficence surely provides a necessary minimal condition for justifying research using human subjects. That is, it is wrong to do research if no good can come of it. Yet the critical question is whether beneficence, by itself, offers a sufficient criterion for deciding that research is ethically acceptable, let alone morally required.

It seems that Bernard would at least have wanted to say that an experiment that may do good is required provided that the person conducting the experiment can come up with no other behavior that could be engaged in at the time that would predictably do as much good. That would bring Bernard into line with some versions of contemporary utilitarian thinking that say that an action is morally required if there is no other action that can do as much good.

THE CONFLICT WITH HIPPOCRATIC MEDICINE

In fact, Bernard has much more serious troubles than any quibbles that might be offered by contemporary utilitarians. He, for instance, in advocating the moral permissibility, even requiredness, of experiments that may do good for mankind, is offering a direct challenge to the Hippocratic tradition in medical ethics. Hippocratic medical ethics, as I use the term, is committed to the core ethical principle found twice in the Hippocratic oath that the physician's ethical duty is to do what will benefit the patient according to the physician's ability and judgment. This view is different from the principle of beneficence in two ways. First, the Hippocratic principle is concerned only with the good of the patient, not with producing good in a more general sense. Second, the Hippocratic principle calls for the physician to decide what is best.

As long as medicine was viewed as a clinical profession—as an art—this Hippocratic principle posed little problem for an ethic of research. Every physician would, if acting ethically, strive to benefit his (or her) patient. If the traditional remedies did not work and the patient's condition was sufficiently grave, the physician could try something new—arguing that a new, untried treatment could be justified in the name of patient welfare. The code of ethics of Thomas Percival, upon which modern Anglo-American professionally articulated physician ethics has been based, made such an appeal saying:

> Whenever cases occur, attended with circumstances not heretofore observed or in which the ordinary modes of practice have been attempted without success, it is for the public good, and in especial degree advantageous to the poor (who, being the most numerous class of society, are the

greatest beneficiaries of the healing art) that new remedies and new methods of chirurgical treatment should be devised.[2]

Innovative treatments, if attempted in the course of clinical care when all standard remedies had failed, could be justified on traditional Hippocratic grounds of trying to benefit the sick. With Bernard, however, an entirely new attitude emerged: the idea of experimentation in a systematic manner for the primary purpose of gaining knowledge. This knowledge would be a potential benefit to mankind in the future, but need not necessarily be intended for the immediate benefit of the subject of the investigation.

What emerged is now often referred to as "non-therapeutic" research, that is, research undertaken on a subject that is not in conjunction with efforts to provide therapy for the subject. Yale pharmacologist Robert Levine has argued with this term, claiming that research, by its very nature, should not be confused with therapy. Research is undertaken to gain knowledge; therapy, what Levine calls "practice," is undertaken solely to benefit a patient. One may, according to Levine's more precise usage, do research on therapeutic procedures, especially on what Levine calls non-validated practices—gather data while administering a drug or procedure—but any given piece of behavior cannot simultaneously be undertaken as a therapeutic practice and as an effort to gain knowledge. It cannot be both simultaneously.[3]

Whether one accepts Levine's terminology or not, once medical researchers began to consider the possibility of doing things to subjects for the purpose of gaining knowledge rather than for the purpose of benefitting them, they collided head-on with their Hippocratic pledge to act always only so as to benefit the patient. If that is taken seriously no Hippocratic physician could ever engage in research in Levine's sense of behavior designed for the purpose of gaining knowledge rather than for the purpose of benefitting the patient.

The World Medical Association has revealed the conflict between the Hippocratic commitment and the beneficence ethic of Bernard. Its 1948 code of ethics, The Declaration of Geneva, is meant to be an updating of the Hippocratic Oath. As such, it is not surprising that it contains the commitment that the physician pledges: "The health of my patient will be my first consideration."[4] If there is any doubt that this prohibits activities undertaken for research purposes, the World Medical Association's International Code of Medical Ethics adopted one year after the Declaration of Geneva, states: "Any act or advice which could weaken physical or mental resistance of a human being may be used only in his interest."[5] Any research procedure that could potentially weaken a patient is excluded.

Once the implications of the Hippocratic tradition for research medicine were realized, however, the World Medical Association had a problem on its hands. It dealt with it essentially by cancelling the Hippocratic oath for research. In 1964 when it wrote its Declaration of Helsinki specifically as a code of ethics for human-subjects research, it had to take explicit note of the two patient-centered commitments already cited. It then went on to carve out a qualification. It said:

> Because it is essential that the results of laboratory experiments be applied to human beings to further scientific knowledge and to help suffering humanity, the World Medical Association has prepared the following recommendations as a guide to each doctor in clinical research.[6]

It then goes on to spell out the ethical requirements for physician participation even in what it calls "non-therapeutic clinical research," that is, research that does not treat the patient as the physician's first consideration and may weaken a human being for reasons unrelated to that person's own interests. Thus, the Hippocratic principle with its sole focus on patient welfare was abandoned, and instead considerations of (full) beneficence were used in order to justify non-therapeutic research.

BERNARD AND THE "PRIMUM NON NOCERE"

There is another way in which the beneficence approach called for by Claude Bernard may be in tension with the traditional ethics of some physicians. Some physicians, when asked what the core of their ethical obligation is, will cite the slogan of physician folk ethics: "First of all, do no harm." Sometimes they even dignify it with the Latin, *primum non nocere*. Yet there is no evidence that this represents an ancient ethical commitment of physicians.[7] Neither is it represented in any modern physician code of ethics. It almost certainly is a minority ethical view even among physicians. Nevertheless to the extent it is an ethical position held even by a minority of physicians, it offers an important ethical challenge to the principle of beneficence as a basis for research medicine.

Exactly what physicians mean when they say that their first or primary duty is to do no harm is unclear. I have elsewhere explored several possibilities.[8] It may simply be a confusing way to express the idea that the physician's actions should be calculated to maximize the net amount of good. If so, it is simply a muddled way of expressing the insight of the principle of beneficence and adds nothing new to the moral deliberation except confusion. It may also be a way of invoking the Catholic doctrine of double effect—that no one should will a direct and intentional evil for another. If that is the meaning, as medical ethicist Albert Jonsen suggests, then the analysis is much more complex.[9]

The most obvious and straightforward meaning derives from the observation that actions may often do both good and harm. It is sometimes held that actively producing harm is morally different from doing good. The two are sometimes distinguished by referring to two moral principles—beneficence and non-maleficence—the principles that actions are right respectively if they produce good or avoid producing evil. The intriguing problem arises when the same action can produce both good and evil. Robin Hood behavior, for example, harms the one from whom resources are taken in order to benefit other persons. A number of writers—including W. D. Ross, William Frankena, and Tom Beauchamp and James Childress[10]—have held that the duty to avoid harming is more stringent than the duty to benefit. That would explain, for example, why it is morally wrong to take the heart, liver, both kidneys, and any other transplantable organs from one person who is of little social usefulness and transplant the harvest into a group of needy, socially useful people who would otherwise die. Giving up one unproductive person to gain several useful lives would seem a good trade if the goal were only to maximize the net amount of good one does. If, however, avoiding harm is a particularly stringent duty—one that takes priority over merely producing good—then the human organ harvesting would be wrong in spite of the increase in net welfare.

The most obvious meaning of the *primum non nocere* maxim is that avoiding harm should get this special priority over simply doing good. That, however, creates a very serious problem for the practice of medicine, especially for research medicine. Carried to its logical extreme the principle that one should first of all avoid doing harm leads to the conclusion that no medical intervention should ever be undertaken. Under such a policy one would miss many opportunities to help people, but at least would avoid harming them. No one carries the priority of non-maleficence to this extreme, however, and that fact challenges the idea that non-maleficence gets any absolute priority over beneficence. Defenders of the moral priority of avoiding harming need to come up with some theory that makes sense out of the idea of a priority without forcing the absurd conclusion that no one should ever act whenever there would be a risk of hurting someone.

Whatever that theory is, some conclude that the priority of not harming at least leads to a rule of thumb that says "when in doubt opt for the course that is likely to do less harm even if it will also probably mean less good will be done as well." In other words the idea that not harming gets priority at least generates a conservative attitude about intervening.

While individuals have every right to opt for such a conservative orientation (or for a more liberal, more pro-interventionist one), the implications for research medicine are horrendous. Many experiments involving human subjects involve trials comparing traditional established treatments with innovative treatments. The research component is the gathering of data to learn which of the two treatments produces better results. The comparison—including a random assignment of the traditional and experimental treatments—is justified on the grounds that the estimated ratio of benefits to harms is comparable in the two cases. The potential benefits of the experimental treatment are likely to be much greater, but, at least in a clinical trial, the harms are likely to be greater as well. It is only when the ratios are in the same range that random assignment is ethical.

If, however, physicians have a moral obligation to give special priority to avoiding harm, then a serious problem occurs. Consider the typical case in which the experimental and traditional treatments have similar expected benefit/harm ratios, but with the potential benefits and harms of the experimental treatment both being much greater. In such a case, if there is a duty to give special priority to avoiding harm, then it would always be immoral to conduct the experimental trial. There would always be an obligation to opt for the more conservative low-risk/low gain option, that is, the traditional treatment. Even if the priority of avoiding harm is not absolute, random clinical trials would be ethically acceptable under the rule of thumb that says "when in doubt avoid harm" only when the benefit-to-harm ratio of the experimental harm is much greater than that of the traditional treatment. That, however, is just the case where randomization would normally be considered immoral. When it seems clear that the expected benefit/harm ratio of the experimental treatment far exceeds that of the traditional treatment, most would conclude that it is immoral to expose the human subject to the risk of getting the traditional treatment.[11] In short, the *primum non nocere*, if it is given its obvious meaning of a priority for avoiding harm over producing benefits, is a conservative ethic that essentially makes even clinical research medicine, that is, research accompanying clinical uses that may benefit the subjects involved, unethical. It is even more disastrous for research not connected with innovative therapies. In those cases essentially no good can come to the patient while harm may come. Even the softer version of the priority for avoiding harm would make such research hard to justify.

Of course, this may simply force us to the conclusion that all or most experimentation really is unethical after all. There are, however, good reasons why a priority for avoiding harm should be rejected. For one, whether a consequence is described as a benefit or a harm is at times dependent upon the exact nature of the characterization of the event, thus different characterizations of the same event would lead to different conclusions about the weights given to various elements. Insofar as we are concerned about consequences at all, it seems much more plausible to strive for maximizing net benefit or benefit/harm ratios rather than giving special weight to harmful consequences. In doing so harm counts no more and no less than benefit. It may be that our considered moral judgments that have sometimes led to giving priority to not harming can be explained by appealing to other ethical principles that take us beyond mere consideration of consequences. It is to these other principles that we now turn.

GOING BEYOND BENEFICENCE

This criticism just discussed comes from those committed to traditional Hippocratic medicine that would insist that interventions be justified on grounds of benefit to the patient or from the holders of the modern deviation of Hippocratic ethics that says that the first obligation of the physician is to avoid harm. Either of these classical physician formulations of their ethical obligation makes research medicine very hard to justify.

THE PROBLEM OF SEVERE HARM TO SUBJECTS

One solution to this problem would be to abandon the Hippocratic, patient-centered focus and the priority for avoiding harm and adopt a straightforward beneficence principle of the sort Bernard or Bentham had in mind. Act in such a way that no alternative behavior is expected to produce greater net benefit. This principle itself, however, creates serious problems. It would seem to justify the proposed harvesting of human organs for transplant in those cases where one person could be sacrificed in order to save many who would otherwise die. Of more immediate concern, the simple version of the utilitarian principle (that is, the version that calculates the utility of each potential act) would seem to justify horrendous experimental interventions on persons without their consent, provided only that the projected benefits exceeded the expected harms (and no alternative way of accomplishing the benefits with less potential harm is envisioned).

The decisive test for this solution to an ethic of research based exclusively on the principle of beneficence was the Nazi research. It is not that the Nazi experiments themselves would obviously have been justified based on beneficence. The harm done to the unwilling subjects was beyond imagination. Moreover, the amount of good that could have come from the experiments is open to doubt. Many have argued that the experiments were so poorly designed that little good could have come out of them and that should have been known in advance. A careful utilitarian taking the simple version of the principle of beneficence might easily show that the harms done, although they were done to a relatively small number, were of such enormous magnitude that they could not have been exceeded by the potential good even if that good could have been applied to billions of people in present and future generations.

While the utilitarian may well be able to show that the Nazi research was not justified on these benefit/harm grounds, that argument misses the point; according to this view it is only a contingent matter whether or not it was justified. Adopting this kind of beneficence-only strategy holds open that in principle someone might be able to design an experiment where horrendous harms done to small numbers of unconsenting subjects would be exceeded by potential benefits to the masses. In order to satisfy the beneficence principle there would have to be no other alternative that would produce greater benefit on balance. That almost surely would mean that subjects would have to be treated as humanely as possible and that the benefits to the masses would truly have to be enormous to justify the taking of life of subjects or subjecting them to severe pain. Provided those conditions were met, however, the simple version of the principle of beneficence would justify inflicting such harm and inflicting it even without the consent of the subjects.

THE NEED FOR OTHER PRINCIPLES

If we want to avoid the implication that we endorse in principle taking the lives of non-consenting subjects or inflicting severe pain on them, some limit must be placed on the principle of beneficence; some other principle must be invoked. This is precisely the position in which the prosecutors in the Nuremberg trials found themselves. They had two options. One was to retreat to the Hippocratic tradition and insist that human subjects be used in medical research only in those cases where the intervention is justified by the potential benefit to the subjects themselves. This move in itself would require moving beyond beneficence. It requires a reason for discriminating between consequences to the subject and consequences to others. It would mean establishing some principle that treats benefits and harms to subjects differently from benefits and harms to others. That in itself would appear to be a violation of the straightforward beneficence principle, which includes consideration of all consequences regardless of the one who bears them. The Hippocratic principle tells the physician to choose the act that produces as much or more net benefit than any other act, but then it adds a crucial qualifier. In calculating benefits and harms, it says, exclude all effects except those that occur to the patient. Thus, some additional principle beyond beneficence is required to justify this limit.

In any case this retreat to the Hippocratic ethic would have solved the problem of sacrificing subjects for social purposes, but the price would have been enormous. The key figures in the trials realized that such an extreme retreat was not necessary. In fact it might well have been unethical as it would have meant foregoing potential benefits for society that could be obtained ethically.

The alternative to retreating to the Hippocratic ethic was to supplement the principle of beneficence with additional requirements. At Nuremberg the awareness of the additional principles needed was quite limited. Principle Two of the Nuremberg Code states the pure and simple version of the beneficence principle: "The experiment should be such as to yield fruitful results for the good of society, unprocurable by other methods or means of study, and not random and unnecessary in nature."[12] It is preceded, however, by a rigorous commitment to the notion of consent. "The voluntary consent of the human subject is absolutely essential."[13]

The authors of the Nuremberg Code saw that they could salvage medical research—even interventions that do not have justification based on potential therapeutic benefit for the subjects themselves—if they subordinated beneficence to an absolute requirement of subject consent.

One possibility is that this is simply a method of replacing the simple version of the beneficence principle with a more complicated way of assuring that the greatest amount of good is likely to be done in research. If subject consent is required, so the argument might go, subjects are much less likely to be the victims of miscalculations of consequences. Operating on the rule of always getting consent may produce greater good in the long run than simply letting researchers calculate whether their research would produce good on balance.

That is the normal first step in the utilitarian's defense of the beneficence principle.[14] Recent normative ethical theory, however, goes much further in attempting to provide a utilitarian basis for the consent requirement. The move just discussed imposes a rule to get consent in the name of trying to assure that each action will most predictably produce good consequences. In fact, however, it seems unlikely that the consent requirement would predictably maximize net good in each research protocol.[15] Surely there must be some situations where violating consent would produce more good. If, for example, an impartial panel were given the authority to judge whether a subject should be experimented upon without his consent and told that it should only authorize such experiments in cases where it was positive that greater good would come than from letting the subject consent, it seems plausible that the principle of beneficence could be served better than by simply operationalizing the consent rule.

The more sophisticated utilitarians have argued over the past two decades that society ought to be governed by certain rules or principles and that the principle of beneficence is only one of these. These people, often called rule utilitarians,[16] argue that social practices should be governed by basic rules or principles that will produce greater good on balance than any other set of rules or principles. They specifically acknowledge the possibility that in a particular instance the greatest good will not result from following the principles. If, for example, requiring respect for autonomy is a basic principle that will tend to produce the greatest good when established as a basic practice in a society, that principle might require consent even if, in a particular instance, more good would come from giving the authority to override consent to an impartial panel.

The rule utilitarians thus supplement the principle of beneficence by adopting a small set of principles each of which will, as a general practice, tend to maximize utility. The writers of the Nuremberg Code may have been incipient rule utilitarians advocating the principle of autonomy and the consent rule derived from it even when in individual cases greater good could come from ignoring the rule. Such an ethic would move beyond the principle of beneficence in the name of trying to produce a set of social arrangements that would produce more good than any alternative set of arrangements.

This rule-utilitarian way of moving beyond beneficence, placed in the hands of a sophisticated philosophical analyst, can probably account for virtually every moral rule that seems plausible. It is not necessarily an accurate account, however, of why those rules were or should be adopted. The critics of the rule utilitarians argue that there is a much more straightforward way of moving beyond beneficence. The rule utilitarians say that there are some basic principles—such as autonomy—upon which a moral society operates because they tend to produce greater good than any alternative set of principles. The critics accept that there is a set of basic principles upon which a society should operate, but question whether those principles are adopted because they produce greater good than any alternative set of principles.

These critics—often called deontologists—might begin with a difficult question for the utilitarian to answer. They might ask why it is morally prima facie right to try to produce good consequences. The response is likely to be something like the following: "At this point we have reached the foundations. Whatever your metaethical theory, it is going to tell you that producing good consequences is a right-making characteristic of actions. If you are a theist, you will hold that God approves of producing good; if you are a rationalist, you will say it is reasonable to produce good; an empiricist will say that it is empirically obvious that producing good is a right-making characteristic of actions. In any case producing good is without question a right-making characteristic." It clearly would not do to offer the argument that the principle of beneficence is a right-making characteristic because it will produce good. That is circular. A defense of the principle of beneficence requires the acceptance that producing good is a right-making characteristic.

Now the deontologist will ask: "Is there any reason why producing good consequences is the only right-making characteristic of actions?" Rather than going through the circumlocution of defending autonomy because it is a principle that will tend to produce good consequences and then defending producing good consequences on the grounds that that is obviously a right-making characteristic of actions (as rule utilitarians must), one could directly maintain that autonomy, like producing good consequences, is a right-making characteristic of actions and therefore is a normative ethical principle.

The test question is to ask oneself why it is that autonomy, for example, is an ethical principle. Is it solely because the autonomy principle will produce better consequences than any alternative principle? If so, then you are a rule utilitarian. If, however, you are prepared to say that the principle of autonomy is an ethical principle simply because respecting the autonomy of individuals is a *prima facie* right-making characteristic *even if it does not tend to produce good consequences*, then you are a deontologist.

The rule utilitarians and rule deontologists share a commitment to a set of principles (or general rules) that specify broad right-making tendencies of actions. Contemporary theorists in medical ethics have demonstrated a substantial convergence around this approach.[17] Moreover, they tend to be able to show considerable agreement on just what principles should be adopted. Every list has a principle of beneficence (perhaps supplemented with a separate principle of non-maleficence). They all have a principle of autonomy (or some surrogate such as the principle of self-determination or liberty). They have a principle of justice as well. I have argued that in addition a full list requires independent principles of promise-keeping and truth-telling as well as a principle that specifies that an action is *prima facie* morally right insofar as it involves avoiding killing of another human being. (Alternatively an action is prima facie wrong insofar as it involves killing another human being.)[18]

These principles taken together do a very fine job of accounting for our moral judgments about research or any other subject in ethics. The principle of avoiding killing, for example, is sufficient to explain why it is morally wrong to take one socially useless citizen and divide his organs among several recipients. So does the principle of autonomy or even the principle of justice, for that matter. Any of these principles does so without relying on the morally suspect idea that avoiding harm takes moral precedence over producing good.

The requirement of informed consent from substantially autonomous persons can be understood as a requirement of the principle of autonomy. This also helps explain why consent is only required from those subjects who are substantially autonomous. The requirement that confidentiality be maintained except under certain circumstances (such as when it is required by law that disclosure be made) can be explained as a requirement of the principle that promises be kept. By the same token the exceptions can be explained by examining the nature of the promise made (or implied) by the researcher. The researcher promises (or should promise) to keep confidences only when the disclosure is not required by law. Other exceptions to the promise of confidentiality should also be specified (there are, for instance, times when breaking confidence is necessary in order to save another party from grave bodily harm), but these details cannot be explored here.

THE PRIORITY OF OTHER PRINCIPLES

The present Department of Health and Human Services regulations governing human-subjects research[19] specify seven criteria for evaluating research:

(1) Risks to subjects are minimized. . . .
(2) Risks to subjects are reasonable in relation to
    anticipated benefits, if any, to subjects,
    and the importance of the knowledge that may reasonably be
    expected to result.
(3) Selection of subjects is equitable.
(4) Informed consent will be sought from each
    prospective subject or the subjects' legally
    authorized representative.
(5) Informed consent will be appropriately documented.
(6) Where appropriate, the research plan makes
    adequate provision for monitoring the data
    collected to insure the safety of subjects.
(7) Where appropriate, there are adequate provisions
    to protect the privacy of subjects and to
    maintain confidentiality of data.

The first two reflect the principle of beneficence—dealing with justification of the risks to the subject and justifying those risks by comparing them to the benefits to the subject and the value of the knowledge to be gained. That principle by itself, however, would justify much too much. Therefore five additional criteria must be met. The next one requires equity in subject selection—rooted in the principle of justice. The next two specify provisions for informed consent—rooted in the principle of autonomy. The next criterion calls for adequate provision for monitoring of data to insure subject safety—a provision logically linked to the principle of beneficence. The final provision assures privacy and confidentiality—a provision I have suggested is grounded in the principle of promise-keeping.

What may not be clear in this list of criteria is what should happen if some of the criteria are satisfied while others are not or if two of the requirements come into conflict. The regulations say that "all of the following requirements" must be satisfied. But what should happen, for example, if one way of conducting the research involves more equitable subject selection, but because of the inconvenience of subject recruitment, will produce somewhat less reliable findings and therefore predictably be somewhat less valuable as a study? It seems unlikely that all seven criteria can be satisfied equally well in all studies.

One strategy is to balance the requirements of the various principles so that that action is morally appropriate that on balance does the best possible job of satisfying all the principles at the same time. Many philosophers have opted for that strategy. In *A Theory of Medical Ethics* I argued against a simple balancing approach.[20] The alternative strategy, of course, assuming that one has more than one ethical principle with which to contend, is to rank order the principles—what John Rawls calls "lexical" ordering, based on the way a dictionary gives an absolute priority to one letter before taking any consideration of the next letter.[21]

Trying to give any one principle absolute priority, however, has been extremely difficult. Rawls is able to lexically order his two principles of justice, but acknowledges that justice must be related to other principles in some fuller theory of ethics. The formula I have defended is one that divides all principles into the consequentialist ones (beneficence and non-maleficence) and the non-consequentialist ones (autonomy, truth-telling, promise-keeping, avoiding killing, and justice). I am prepared to accept a balancing strategy among the non-consequentialist principles. Thus truth telling and avoiding killing are *prima facie* co-equal in their priority. I am also prepared to accept such a balancing strategy among the two consequentialist principles. Thus avoiding harm (non-maleficence) does not have any special standing in comparison with producing good (beneficence) as I have already argued.

The innovation, however, is that between consequentialist and non-consequentialist principles the non-consequentialist ones must take priority. They are jointly lexically ordered over any consideration of consequences. The non-consequentialist principles must be satisfied in full before any consideration of consequences can come into play.

This is consistent with the widely held ethical position that no amount of good consequences would justify killing a subject for research purposes. Likewise, the mere consideration of benefits that may be produced if consent is overridden cannot justify violation of autonomy. No amount of anticipated good justifies overriding the principles of autonomy or justice or avoiding killing.

In assessing the ethics of research this means that the criteria based on the non-consequentialist principles must be satisfied first. Once these are satisfied, then one can move on to consider questions of benefit and harm. Of course, even if the other principles are satisfied, a proposed piece of research would have to offer benefits that outweigh the projected risks to the subjects, and the risks to the subjects would have to be minimized (or else some other approach would offer greater net benefit). What is critical, however, is that these benefit/harm considerations come into play only when the other conditions are met. We move beyond beneficence in such a way that the non-consequentialistic ethical principles take precedence over it. It is in this sense that the DHHS regulations can call for all the criteria to be satisfied.

THE IMPLICATIONS OF MOVING BEYOND BENEFICENCE

Beneficence then is a minimally necessary condition for ethically acceptable research, but the other ethical principles are also necessary conditions. In fact, they take priority over mere production of good consequences. Never can beneficence—the anticipation of good to be done—justify compromising any of the non-consequentialistic principles. If beneficence is (only) a minimally necessary condition in evaluating the ethics of research, there are direct implications for several specific issues.

The Subjective Element in Calculating Benefits and Harms

A mental estimate of the potential benefits and harms of each research project using human subjects will be essential. This will require determination of the benefits and harms to the individual subject as well as to society. For any given subject, however, the potential benefits and burdens may be evaluated quite differently. A week's hospitalization or a day's nausea or a moment's pain from a needle mean different things to different people. The risks to the subject must be reasonable in relation to the anticipated benefits to the subject and the importance of the knowledge that may reasonably be expected. That judgment, however, requires very subjective assessments of how bad the potential harms, burdens, and inconveniences to the subject are as well as how beneficial possible goods may be. In some cases even deciding whether an effect is a benefit or a harm will be a matter of subjective interpretation. An extra day of stay in a hospital may be a burden for one subject, but a benefit for another.

This is one of the reasons why the layperson must be an active participant in the research process. Without his or her active involvement it is literally impossible to know what the potential benefits and harms will be for a given case of human-subject experimentation. Thus without active input from the patient or other subject it will be impossible to determine whether the risks to the subject are reasonable in comparison with the potential benefits to the subject and the importance of the knowledge to be gained.

ASSESSING RESEARCH DESIGN AND SCIENTIFIC MERIT

By the same token assessing the importance of the knowledge to be gained also requires evaluative judgment based on some framework of values. In the first analysis deciding whether a protocol is likely to produce an answer to the research question posed and produce it as reliably as is feasible— assessing the research design—seems to be a purely objective, scientific matter, perhaps best left to a panel of experts in statistics, research methodology, and the specific research area under consideration rather than to an institutional review board or a layperson. Even that, as we shall see momentarily, must be questioned. Even if assessment of research design is a scientific question, however, determining the merit of the research is surely not.

Deciding how important it is to know an answer to a scientific question is fundamentally not a scientific problem. It is a discussion in which any person can participate. In fact specialists in medical research, especially in medical research of the type being assessed, can be expected to have systematically atypical assessments of the value of the knowledge to be gained. One would expect those who have given their lives to pursuing particular research questions to be atypical in their assessment of how important it is to answer them. They probably would normally overvalue the knowledge being pursued, but they might undervalue it. In any case there is good reason to expect that their assessments will not be typical. Insofar as the question is a particular subject's participation in the research, that subject's personal, subjective assessment of the importance of the knowledge to be gained will be essential. That is why as part of the consent process each subject must be told the purpose of the study. For any proposed research each individual subject has to form a judgment about whether the objectives are beneficial. Some objectives may be viewed as important by researchers, but trivial or even detrimental by some subjects. Only with active participation of the subject will the comparison of risks and benefits be possible.

Insofar as the question arises at a more general level—at the time when the department or institution is deciding whether to approve the research, individual subject variation is not as relevant and may not be assessable in any case. It is crucial, however, to have an assessment of the importance of the knowledge to be gained from the point of view of the institution's value system as well as that of the broader society. It is for this reason that review panels must be given a chance to evaluate the importance of the knowledge being pursued and that panels dealing with questions of scientific merit should be as removed as possible from the special value commitments of researchers.

Even assessing research design raises unexpected problems of subjectivity. A wide range of judgments made in assessing research design are inherently non-scientific. Deciding what confidence level is acceptable will be critical in deciding whether the sample size is sufficiently large, yet that is fundamentally a non-scientific choice. Deciding which methods best test the hypotheses and which concepts best formulate the questions are likewise matters dependent upon non-scientific choices. It is inherent in the judgments about conducting research that these evaluative judgments must be made.

THE MINIMAL RISK LIMIT

These observations about the subjective element in assessing benefits and harms and in assessing research design and scientific merit are directly implied in the beneficence principle. The treatment of the beneficence principle as a minimal condition which is subordinated to non-consequentialist principles is seen in several other aspects of the key documents dealing with human-subjects research. One example is the concept of minimal risk, which is appealed to at a number of points. For research to be reviewed by expedited review (review by less than the full IRB), for example, it must involve no more than minimal risk. Research involving prisoners, children, pregnant women, and fetuses must be assessed to determine whether risk is minimal, and if that condition is not met research is either prohibited or controlled more rigorously.

Once again, however, the judgment that risk is minimal is subjective. "Minimal risk" is defined as:

> risks of harm anticipated in the proposed research are not greater, considering probability and magnitude, than those ordinarily encountered in daily life or during the performance of routine physical or psychological examinations or tests.[22]

Not only is this judgment of minimal harm subjective; it is also hard to square it with the principle of beneficence. If the only ethical consideration in human-subjects research were producing good (and avoiding harm), then a minimal risk to a subject would be justified by a slightly above minimal benefit to the subject or society. By the same token, however, a proportionally larger risk to the subject would be justified by a proportionally larger potential benefit.

A limit related to minimal risk is imposed in those cases where the subject cannot consent and greater risk is not justified by potential benefits to the subject. Such a limitation requires a moral recognition that benefits and harms cannot be traded off among different people at least not beyond a rather small amount or not without the consent of the one exposed to the harm. Only principles other than beneficence can possibly explain such a restriction. The most obvious principle is the principle of justice, which is concerned with the distribution rather than the amount of benefit and harm.

The concept of minimal or limited risk to the subject is applied even in cases where subjects are competent and could give an informed consent to very great risk. The important case would be a research proposal involving severe harm (or extreme risk of serious harm) to a competent subject. Assuming the protocol was for an important purpose and provided for impeccable criteria to assure that the subject was competent and not unduly coerced to consent, would research be permitted that involved deliberate amputation of a limb or a one-in-twenty risk of death solely for research purposes? Most review boards and funding agencies would probably disapprove, yet such research might be justified on grounds of potential new benefits and allowed by the principle of autonomy.

The opposition might be based on pure paternalism, a concern that persons should be protected against choices that jeopardize their own interests. It is not clear, however, that such a choice would violate the subject's interest. Depending upon how the subject is compensated and how much personal satisfaction he or she receives from contributing to humankind, the participation may be a net benefit even considering only his or her own welfare.

Even if it were not, it is hard to see how the principle of beneficence could lead to a decision to oppose the research provided that the benefits to society outweighed the harms, however great, to the subject. If there is a basis for opposition, it must be on grounds that are neither paternalistic nor purely consequentialistic. The most plausible grounds would be that participation would violate the institution's or society's own commitments. Insofar as a serious risk of death was involved, opposition might be based on the principle of avoiding killing human beings. Even if the cause is a good one, such killing is wrong, at least *prima facie*, according to this principle. If the harm is merely one of, say, amputation, some other basis would have to be found for our objection. Permitting such research might, for example, be seen as permitting an unjust rearrangement of the benefits and burdens in the society, or it might simply be aesthetically unacceptable for the institution or the society to be part of such a major deliberate wrongdoing (even if greater good was expected to come of it).

In spite of the principle of beneficence, an institution is normally seen as justified in endorsing research only when the risks to the subject are relatively comparable to the benefits to the subject (taking into account probability and magnitude). This is true regardless of the potential benefits to society. This means, for example, that in a randomized clinical trial randomization will be acceptable only if the benefit-harm ratios of the treatment arms are more or less similar. As soon as one treatment arm's ratio gets out of line a reassessment will be required. If the ratio is much lower, offering that arm will be seen as unacceptable. As we shall see in later chapters this creates enormous problems as these benefit and harm projections begin to change as the result of preliminary data. It also creates serious problems if one individual subject's subjective assessment of benefits and harms varies considerably. It may make participation inappropriate for certain atypical subjects although appropriate for more typical ones—a matter that can be dealt with easily if the subject is an active participant adequately informed of the current state of data. It may, however, also make participation in a randomization appropriate for these atypical subjects although it would be inappropriate for the normal candidates. Although this may appear to make life difficult for researchers, it may actually offer a tremendous opportunity to recruit subjects ethically (as we shall see in chapter nine's discussion of the "semi-randomized clinical trial").

Evaluating Risk-Free Research

One issue related to the subordination of the beneficence principle arose especially in conjunction with the regulations from the Department of Health, Education, and Welfare in the 1970s.[23] Those regulations began by saying that an institutional review board was to assess any proposed research governed by the regulations and determine whether human subjects were placed at risk. If they were, then the proposal was to be reviewed to assure that:

(1) The risks to the subject are so outweighed by the sum of the benefit to the subject and the importance of the knowledge to be gained as to warrant a decision to allow the subject to accept these risks;

(2) The rights and welfare of any such subjects will be adequately protected; and

(3) Legally effective informed consent will be obtained by adequate and appropriate methods. . . . [24]

It makes sense to apply the first criterion (to determine whether the risks to the subject are justified) only in those cases where subjects are at risk. The critical question is why, in the light of the arguments presented here, research should be assessed to assure that the rights of the subject are protected and that there is a legally effective informed consent only in those cases where subjects are at risk. This version of the regulations provided the paradoxical combination of an explicit recognition that considerations other than benefits and harms are at stake (by imposing two additional conditions beyond benefit/harm assessment) and simultaneously providing for consideration of those other conditions only when subjects were at risk. It should be clear that important ethical issues can be at stake even when subjects are placed at no risk. The right to confidentiality, for example, could be infringed. The right to consent could be violated, even if the subject were not at risk.

It might be argued that no subject would care about consenting if he or she were not at any risk for harm. A little reflection, however, reveals cases where consent could be critical. One of the elements of an informed consent is information about the purpose of the research. Subjects may be asked to participate in research the purpose of which is highly objectionable to them. Studies of medical records to compare race with intelligence or to develop information about ethically suspect procedures such as abortion would be examples. Clandestine video-taping of patients in their hospital beds may subject patients to no harm, but still be objectionable to many. Subjects could object even though they were not at risk.

It might be argued that in these cases subjects really are at risk—at risk of having their confidences violated or their wishes overridden. In that sense every subject of every imaginable so-called risk-free study is really at potential risk. If that were one's understanding of risk, then, however, no possible study could be found to be "risk-free." Every study would go though the initial step of determining whether subjects were at risk and would be found to have some risks.

The textual evidence is quite clear that this was not the intended meaning in the old DHEW regulations. It made a distinction between research that was "risk-free" in the sense of not exposing the subjects to physical, psychological, or social injury and research that was not. But then only in cases where such risks occurred were the rights of the subject protected by review mechanisms, and only in those cases was consent required. The priority on non-consequentialist principles was stood on its head. Only in cases where risk of injury was at stake were the rights of subjects to be protected.

EXCEPTIONS FOR RESEARCH IN THE DHHS GUIDELINES

On January 26, l981, new regulations on the protection of human subjects went into effect.[25] They dropped the requirement that distinguishes between risk-free and risky research. In its place, however, two new categories of research were created. One involved research for which expedited review—often by only one institutional review board member—was sufficient. It involves research where subjects are exposed to no more than minimal risk and the only involvement of human subjects is in one or more of ten listed activities such as collection of small samples of blood or study of existing data. Since such research normally involves few if any moral problems the expedited review makes sense. What is important is that someone sensitive to possible moral questions of consent, justice, privacy, etc., looks at every study.

The second new category creates more of a problem. It is research that is exempt from any review. Six categories of research are completely exempt from the federally mandated review process. These include studies in educational settings, using educational tests, interviews, survey research, etc., when certain additional conditions pertaining to sensitive subject matter and confidentiality are met.

The problem here is that, provided research meets the conditions specified, none of the ethical requirements—equitable subject selection, protection of confidentiality, and assurance of adequate consent—must be met. Research could be conducted, for example, using existing medical records to study whether hormonal levels differ in males and females for the purpose of defending a thesis that males and females are fundamentally different in certain characteristics that have bearing on employment or personality or educational achievement. Provided the individuals whose records were being studied could not be identified, such research would be exempt from any review. Even though many subjects might seriously object to the purpose of the study, they would not be given a chance to consent or refuse consent to have their records used for this purpose. There would not even be an institutional review board examination of the study to see what rights of subjects need protection. Once again because the risk of injury appears virtually non-existent, basic rights rooted in the non-con-sequentialist principles are violated.

It might be argued that subjects in such a study really are at risk. They could be discriminated against as a result of the impact of the study. According to the existing regulations that makes no difference. The research is exempt. More fundamentally, however, even if subjects concede that they are not at risk for such harm, they might want to have the opportunity to refuse to participate. The appearance of lack of risk once again has suppressed the consideration of the ethics of studies on grounds of non-con-sequentialist principles.

Exclusions of Long-Term Social Risks

Most puzzling for the application of the principle of beneficence as minimal condition for ethically acceptable research is the DHHS treatment of long-term public policy risks:

> The IRB should not consider possible long-range effects of applying knowl-edge gained in the research (for example, the possible effects of the research on public policy) as among those research risks that fall within the purview of its responsibility.[26]

It is hard to know precisely what the regulation writers had in mind here. If one of the long-range effects of applying the knowledge gained is that thousands of lives may be saved by the drug being tested, is the IRB to exclude this fact and consider only the short-term benefits and harms? Surely not.

Presumably what the writers were trying to exclude was consideration of more subtle long-term effects, especially detrimental ones. For example, if a new genetic engineering technology under study might one day be used in some evil scheme to reshape the human personality, that would be a per-vasive long-range effect but extremely difficult for the review panel to assess. It is reported that the regulation writers believed that the panels were not in a good position to assess these kinds of effects and therefore tried to exclude them. In the process, however, they come dangerously close to saying that panels can consider the good effects—like curing disease—but not the bad ones. In that situation the principle of beneficence is easy to satisfy.

If the IRB is not permitted to assess these long-range bad effects, then someone surely must. Otherwise even the minimal condition of the principle of beneficence is not met. Even if it is met, however, it should be clear that other, more critical, moral conditions must be met for research to be acceptable. It must satisfy, first and foremost, a set of ethical requirements based on consideration of non-consequentialist principles such as autonomy and justice. To these considerations we now turn.

CHAPTER THREE

The Principle of Autonomy: The Foundation for Informed Consent

If we are to move beyond exclusively focusing on beneficence, we need to determine what other ethical principles govern research using human subjects and how these principles can be weighed against each other when in conflict. The study of the principle or principles that justify informed consent is not only important in itself. It also provides an excellent illustration of the controversy over whether beneficence is sufficient in itself to ground ethics. If we must move beyond beneficence, one important additional principle will be the principle of autonomy. A good place to look at the principle of autonomy is in the notion of informed consent. It is very difficult, as we shall see in this chapter, to ground the informed consent requirement in beneficence. A much more firm foundation is provided by adding the principle of autonomy to our list of ethical principles.

As we saw in the last chapter, Department of Health, Education, and Welfare regulations governing human-subjects research in the mid-1970s required local review of all biomedical and behavioral research on human subjects supported under grants and contracts from the department to determine whether subjects would be placed at risk and, "if risk is involved," whether "legally effective informed consent will be obtained by adequate and appropriate methods."[1] The logical implication is that informed consent of human subjects, insofar as it was mandated by DHEW regulations, was subordinated to and derived from the goal of protecting human subjects from risk, that is, from the principle of beneficence. That places informed consent on an inadequate base.

My objective is to analyze the philosophical foundations of informed consent, articulating three theories of informed consent and the implications of those theories for public policy. Informed consent cannot be derived solely from the notion of avoiding risks and/or maximizing good consequences, but must have an independent philosophical foundation. That foundation, so I shall argue, is the principle of autonomy—of self-determination. After exploring three major competing theories of informed consent, I shall then examine the implications for deciding how much information ought to be transmitted for consent to be informed. Finally I shall trace some of the policy implications first for informed consent from competent, non-institutionalized subjects and then for subjects who are legally incompetent, institutionalized, or both.

I. THREE THEORIES OF INFORMED CONSENT

Although this is a discussion of the philosophical grounding of informed consent in a research setting, a good case can be made that the same principles apply to consent in routine clinical contexts as well.[2] Thus this is, in reality, an exploration of the role of the principle of autonomy in consent in either context.

The notion of consent is a modern one. Qualifying consent with the adjectives "free" and "informed" is even more modern, yet surely central to the contemporary discussion.[3] Nonetheless, to develop a theory of the foundations of consent it is essential to place the concept in a historical context.

A. THE PATIENT-BENEFIT THEORY OF INFORMED CONSENT

Traditionally experimentation in medicine was an integral part of the treatment of the patient. The Hippocratic authors placed medicine on a more naturalistic footing than it had stood previously. In works such as *The Sacred Disease* the Hippocratic corpus demystifies diseases such as epilepsy.[4] The author argues with regard to epilepsy, which had at the time been interpreted as being caused by sacred powers: "It is not, in my opinion, any more divine or more sacred than other diseases, but has a natural cause, and its supposed divine origin is due to men's inexperience, and their wonder at its peculiar character."[5]

In spite of the fact that Hippocratic and Galenic medicine viewed medical problems as natural phenomena, these traditions did not rationalize and systematize medical experimentation as we know it. This did not happen until modern times. The Hippocratic physician would try out new remedies, but always in the context of treating a patient when routine therapies were not successful. It was not until well into the modern period that medical experimentation was undertaken in the sense of systematically designed research for the purpose of gaining medical knowledge. It is in part for this reason that the notion of consent is absent from the Hippocratic tradition.

The ethic of the Hippocratic physician was (and to some extent still is) rooted in a special set of norms. According to Ludwig Edelstein the deontological (ethical) writings of the Hippocratic corpus reflect the philosophical, religious, and scientific views of the Pythagorean cult.[6] The dominating ethical norm is, as we have seen, that the physician's duty is to do what will benefit the patient according to his ability and judgment.[7]

Although modern physicians may never even have read the original Hippocratic oath, the ethical norms are ones with which they are likely to be comfortable. The World Medical Association in 1949 adopted an International Code of Medical Ethics which includes an updated version of the patient-benefitting principle: "Under no circumstances is a doctor permitted to do anything that would weaken the physical or mental resistance of a human being except from strictly therapeutic or prophylactic indications imposed in the interest of his patient." It is generally thought that the Hippocratic oath may be rather platitudinous. It is usually not recognized how controversial the principle itself is.[8] For our purposes the primary implication is that all physician activity, including medical experimentation that is not undertaken for the benefit of the patient, ought to be forbidden.[9]

Although the requirement of informed consent is not traditional in Hippocratic medicine, it is possible to justify such a requirement on patient-benefitting grounds. Indeed, if we recognize that judgments about what is beneficial to a particular patient will vary from patient to patient depending upon the particular norms and values of that person, a strong case can be made that informing patients of treatment alternatives so that they can participate in, or even control, the decision-making process will increase the likelihood that patient benefits will be maximized. Especially in cases of research related to therapeutic procedures,[10] that is, research in which pursuit of knowledge is associated with procedures with potential benefit to the patient, patients might plausibly maximize benefits by choosing between more conservative, standard therapies and experimental therapies on the basis of their own inclination to take chances and their faith in technological innovation.[11] Thus even in classical Hippocratic ethics informed consent may have an important place.

The decisive case for testing the relationship between patient benefit and informed consent ought to be the special situation where someone (usually the physician) believes that getting patient consent will do harm to the patient rather than produce benefit. Testing an experimental cancer drug on a terminally ill patient who does not know his diagnosis or prognosis is a good example. If informed consent is a derivative principle designed to insure patient benefit, then whenever getting consent would do more harm than good it ought to be waived. This exemption is explicit in the 1971 FDA regulations for use of an investigational new drug. Consent is to be obtained except where the investigators "deem it not feasible or, in their professional judgment, contrary to the best interest of such human beings" (i.e., the subjects).[12] It is implied in the December 1, 1971, version of the DHEW Guidelines. Citing the important Halushka v. University of Saskatchewan case, the guidelines specify that:

Where an activity involves therapy, diagnosis, or management, and a professional/patient relationship exists, it is necessary "to recognize that each patient's mental and emotional condition is important . . . and that in discussing the element of risk, a certain amount of discretion must be employed consistent with full disclosure of fact necessary to any informed consent."[13]

The draft regulations as revised and published in the *Federal Register* October 9, 1973,[14] and the final regulations as published May 30, 1974,[15] had no such exclusion. There are two possible explanations. First, the drafters of the regulations may have continued in their commitment to patient benefit, but held that consent will, on balance, be a practice which is patient-benefitting in the sense of protecting them from risk even in those cases where researchers believe that the patient would be benefitted more by not being told.[16] If physicians were not capable of perceiving what would benefit the patient—in terms of the patient's own values—or what the patient's response to the request for consent would be, then the consent should be obtained even if, in the physician's judgment, it might do harm.[17] Alternatively they may have held that informed consent is so fundamental to the subject's rights that it must be retained even in cases where the physician (rightly) perceives that it might do more harm than good.[18]

We are left with a confusion in the 1974 DHEW guidelines. Consent is only required in cases where subjects have been found to be at risk, implying that consent is somehow inherently linked with and subordinated to the primary goal of protecting patients from harm. On the other hand the researcher and the local committee are not permitted to waive consent on grounds of net patient-benefit.

More doubt is cast on the adequacy of the patient-benefit grounds for informed consent when one realizes that the patient-benefit principle tradition in medicine would rule out entirely all experiments unrelated to therapeutic interventions, that is, experiments designed to gain knowledge useful to society, but not involving procedures with risks justified on patient-benefitting grounds alone. It is clear that any physician who holds to the principles of the Hippocratic oath cannot participate in any so-called non-therapeutic research. To do so would be to act other than strictly for the benefit of his patient.

The standard of the Hippocratic ethic, however, is the standard of a private, professional group. The ethical principles of private groups, including medical groups, ought to be of minimal importance for public policy or for public groups such as the National Commission for the Protection of Human Subjects. It is the purpose of such bodies to determine an ethically acceptable basis for human experimentation whether or not that basis is consistent with the ethical view of any such private groups. Nevertheless, it is of interest that the medical profession itself has abandoned its sole commitment to patient benefit when it considers non-therapeutic experimentation. In 1954, five years after its general reaffirmation of the patient-benefitting principle as the only grounds under which a physician could do anything to weaken the physical or mental resistance of a human being, the World Medical Association adopted its "Principles for Those in Research and Experimentation." It clearly approves research on healthy subjects, apparently contradicting its earlier pledge limiting physician actions to patient well-being. By 1962 in the Declaration of Helsinki, the World Medical Association explicitly adopted a principle approving of research independent of therapeutically justified interventions "because it is essential that the results of laboratory experiments be applied to human beings to further scientific knowledge and to help suffering humanity."[19] The American Medical Association has similarly approved of such research implying that it too has abandoned the Hippocratic or patient-benefitting ethic as its decisive norm.[20]

What is of primary importance to public policy, however, is not the norms of private groups, including professional groups, but publicly legitimated and accepted ethical standards. In one sense a public commission's task is the protection of human subjects. Clearly the easiest way to protect human subjects would be to ban all non-therapeutic research. Consent might be justified for therapeutic experiments on patient-benefitting grounds, but it is not clear that consent should always be required even in those experiments. It would be required when, and only when, patients would be more likely to benefit by giving consent.

The National Commission and by now most reasonable people in our society seem to agree that at least some experimentation independent of therapy is acceptable. If that is the case, however, the sole task of relevant public policy cannot be the protection of human subjects. Likewise, the sole foundation of informed consent cannot be patient-benefit. In fact when patients consent to non-therapeutic experimentation, and to much therapeutic experimentation as well, consent seems to function more to cancel the implicit obligation of the physician that he or she will strive only to benefit the patient (and protect him from harm). Logically, if consent functions to waive the obligations of the norm of patient-benefit, it cannot itself be grounded in patient-benefit.

Since the logical implication of the patient-benefitting principle—that research can be done only for the benefit of the individual patient/subject—is strongly counter-intuitive, that awareness may be sufficient to reject the patient-benefitting principle as the foundation of informed consent.

The principle itself, however, implies an even better reason. One should ask why it is that physicians or others would feel a duty to act only so as to benefit the patient and protect him or her from harm. It seems the most plausible answer is that the individual human being (who is sometimes in the patient role) is seen as an autonomous entity with special claims against the rest of us—claims normally called rights. This awareness that the individual human is uniquely endowed with rights is variously expressed in the Western tradition by saying that humans were created in the image of God (Genesis), are to be treated as an end and never only as a means (Kant), or simply that they are endowed by their Creator with certain inalienable rights. If, however, the individual person is always to be treated as an end and never only as a means, it must mean more than that simply others must avoid taking risks with that individual. To be a person is to be an autonomous individual, the possessor of rights and of the freedom of self-determination. After all, "autonomous" means self-governing. Persons are, at minimum, the possessors of what philosophers call negative rights or liberty rights—rights that protect individual freedom of choice and action insofar as such acts do no harm to others. These rights are grounded in a principle of autonomy rather than beneficence.

This notion of the human as an autonomous individual who is the possessor of rights is not explicit in the patient-benefitting Hippocratic tradition. In fact, the explicit notion of individual rights is, like the principle of informed consent, uniquely modern. It is understandable that modern medical professionals who remain Hippocratic in their ethic would tend to link consent to risks and benefits for the patient. For those more explicitly committed to individual rights, however, the Hippocratic view limited to benefits and risks to the patient will be an inadequate foundation for the patient-physician relationship. It will be even less adequate for the relationship between researcher and subject.

B.   THE SOCIAL-BENEFIT THEORY OF INFORMED CONSENT

If it seems implausible that the primary purpose of informed consent is to protect patients against risk—although it may in some instances function in this way—some may find its purpose in the more generally accepted ethical theory of utilitarianism. According to this view, as articulated by Bentham, Mill, and others,[21] that course of action is right which produces the greatest good for the greatest number. Experimentation would be justified according to this view if, all things considered, more good than harm came from the experiment and as much net good came from the experiment as from any other plausible course of action. Holders of this view are sophisticated in recognizing that good cannot be limited to economic considerations. Aesthetic, cultural, religious, and psychological goods and harms would have to be taken into account. Depriving a small group of subjects of their liberty would not necessarily be justified by good to a great number of others if that one counted the deprivation as a very grave harm.

If non-therapeutic experiments are to be justified at all, there almost has to be some element of social benefit included in the justification. As long as experimenting in medicine was in the context of patient care, that is, when experiments were linked to interventions that were therapeutic in intent, social benefits of the research were ancillary. With the modern period, however, when rational design of research in the pursuit of knowledge gave independent grounds for experimenting, benefits to others became significant and at the same time introduced a potential conflict with the benefit-to-patient norm.

It is often not realized that systematically designed experimentation is a modern phenomenon: Experimental medicine is often dated from William Harvey's publication of his studies of animal circulation in 1628.[22] While this work exemplifies research for the pursuit of knowledge, even this did not involve systematically controlled research exposing human subjects to such risks as double-blind placebo administration. Systematic investigation of this kind is a nineteenth- and even more a twentieth-century phenomenon.

By the beginning of the nineteenth century research for the good of society rather than the individual patient began to be defended. Thomas Percival was asked by the trustees of the Manchester Infirmary to prepare a code of ethical conduct for physicians to help them overcome an internal dispute. (The Code, which was published in 1803, has become the foundation of Anglo-American physician ethics.) In the document Percival is explicit in justifying medical experimentation on broader public-benefit grounds.[23]

There is not any hint of a patient-consent requirement, but there must be previous consultation with "the gentlemen of the faculty." Given the context of the tensions at the Manchester Infirmary at the time, it is plausible to see this consultation as serving more general social purposes, including the protection of the hospital's image, as well as making sure that the experimentation is "for the public good, and in especial degree advantageous for the poor."

As seen earlier, in chapter 2, for Claude Bernard, the father of modern medical experimentation, the justification of experimentation in terms of the general good goes even further. In his 1865 *Introduction to the Study of Experimental Medicine* he boldly claims that "Christian morals forbid only one thing, doing ill to one's neighbor. So, among the experiments that may be tried on man, those that can only harm are forbidden, those that are innocent are permissible, and those that may do good are obligatory."[24]

The question remains, if the underlying justification of medical experimentation is that it will produce good social consequences on balance, what is the place of informed consent? If maximizing good consequences were the only relevant consideration, it seems reasonable that often more research could be done more efficiently if the consent requirement were eliminated.

There is one justification for the consent requirement, however, even on social-benefit grounds. It may be that a general policy of research for social good without patient or subject consent would soon create public suspicion and severe handicap for the research enterprise. Subjects would resist situations where experiment was likely. A requirement that all subjects must give consent would assure laypeople that they would not be unknowing subjects of medical research. The general consent rule might simply be a clever way of promoting long-run social utility.[25]

A test case would be an experiment which by its very nature could not be done with consent, for example, certain psychological studies of perception requiring the use of deception. Under these circumstances no good could come if consent were obtained, while some good might come if the research were permitted under controlled non-consent circumstances. This social-utility theory of consent underlay the 1974 DHEW regulations that permit waiving of the consent requirement when "use of either of the primary procedures for obtaining informed consent would surely invalidate objectives of considerable immediate importance."[26] Even the current DHHS regulations include a set of conditions under which consent may be waived.[27] One of the conditions for waiving consent, however, poses an intriguing problem. One requirement for waiving consent is that such a waiver "not adversely affects the rights and welfare of the subjects."[28] If, however, one of the rights of the subject is the right to self-determination based on an adequately informed consent and at least some subjects would want to know if deception is part of the research design, then logically no proposed consent waiver could ever meet the specified conditions.

There is some evidence that the original introduction of consent for research in the nineteenth century had as one of its purposes the preservation of the research for the social good which would come. In 1822 William Beaumont began his famous experiments on gastric physiology. His work was made possible because one Alexis St. Martin suffered an accidental shotgun wound leaving a fistula (a direct opening) to the stomach. St. Martin signed a written contract with Beaumont agreeing to be his "covenant servant" for one year.[29] St. Martin was destitute and destined to be deported as an alien unless he could find some way to support himself. His agreement with Beaumont was the solution. Its quality is primitive by late twentieth-century standards. Being a binding agreement it seems in part designed to guarantee that once Dr. Beaumont had invested in the subject, St. Martin would continue with him until the results could be demonstrated to his colleagues.[30]

While there are instances where the consent seems to function to serve the general social welfare rather than protect the patient, for the most part that does not seem to be its primary purpose. In fact while, in contrast to the patient-benefitting principle, the principle of social benefit legitimates non-therapeutic research, it seems to legitimate too much. According to the principle, research that would on balance serve the general welfare would have to be done. Only in cases where the consent facilitated the research would the consent be necessary.

It is the social-benefits principle which, together with some strangely ethnocentric values, led to the Nazi experiments and the decisive challenge to the *bonum commune* defense of medical experimentation.[31] It became clear at Nuremberg as never before that fundamental human rights were at stake in non-therapeutic research justified on the grounds of the greater good for society.

C. THE SELF-DETERMINATION THEORY OF INFORMED CONSENT

If maximizing social benefits leads to unacceptable violation of the rights of the individual subject, the drafters of the Nuremberg Code had two options. They could return to the older Hippocratic formula insisting the research be undertaken only when it is justifiable in terms of benefit to the patient/ subject. Alternatively they could hold to the legitimacy of research for the good of the community and control against excesses by articulating some limiting principle. The authors chose the latter course. The second principle of Nuremberg makes clear that social benefit has not been abandoned.[32] But informed consent is introduced as the first principle. It states that "the voluntary consent of the human subject is absolutely essential."[33] We are led to an inescapable conclusion. Anyone who imposes an informed-consent requirement on medical research for a reason other than the instrumental value that consent might have in furthering research for the common good must recognize that individual subjects have claims against the society, claims so strong we call them "rights." There must be rights of the individual, who has standing even against the claim that the greater good would be served if those rights were compromised. The rights we are referring to here are liberty rights, rights grounded in the principle of autonomy.

This should not sound strange at least for one steeped in Anglo-American political philosophy. Americans have learned that all are endowed by their Creator with certain inalienable rights including life, liberty, and the pursuit of happiness. The Constitutional guarantee to due process before deprivation of liberty cannot be sacrificed simply because the good of the community would be served.

Although informed consent may, upon occasion, promote benefits to the patient and/or benefits to society, it is clear that its primary purpose stands over against these consequentialist objectives. The principle of autonomy gives the individual certain claims that cannot be overridden simply because it would be in the interests of either society or the individual to do so. When persons consent to be exposed to certain risks for the good of a broader social agenda, they are waiving certain of the claims they have to be protected from risks that others may want to impose because they serve society's purposes. It is the principle of autonomy that makes informed consent necessary for all invasions of the body or even invasions of one's privacy. The principle of autonomy—and its derivative right to self-determination—provides an independent foundation for the informed-consent requirement, a foundation much more solid than the justifications of informed consent that occasionally can be plausibly but not conclusively derived from concern over protection of the individual against risk or protection of the society by protecting the larger research enterprise. It is because of this autonomy foundation that consent giving can be seen as a negotiation of a contract.

There is strong legal evidence that this autonomy-based theory of informed consent is the true philosophical foundation of the consent requirement. This was not always the case in American jurisprudence, however. As late as 1871[34] and again in 1895[35] major court opinions dealing with experimentation omitted any requirement for consent. But in 1914 Justice Cardozo articulated forcefully the patient's right to self-determination as the basis for surgery:

> Every human being of adult years and sound mind has a right to determine what shall be done with his own body; and a surgeon who performs an operation without his patient's consent commits an assault, for which he is liable in damages. . . . This is true except in cases of emergency where the patient is unconscious and where it is necessary to operate before consent can be obtained. . . .[36]

The self-determination principle was reaffirmed as the foundation of that consent in Natanson v. Kline in 1960 where Justice Schroeder argued:

> Anglo-American law starts with the premise of thorough-going self-determination. It follows that each man is considered to be master of his own body, and he may, if he be of sound mind, expressly prohibit the performance of life-saving surgery, or other medical treatment.[37]

The principle of consent was applied to experimentation as opposed to routine treatment in Fortner v. Koch[38] in 1935.

There is some evidence that the authors of the 1974 DHEW regulations recognized that informed consent as well as other rights are independent of the question of risks and benefits to subject and society. Whenever review was mandated, review committees had three substantive tasks: (a) to determine whether the risks to the subject are so outweighed by the sum of the benefit to the subject and the importance of the knowledge to be gained as to warrant a decision to allow the subject to accept these risks; (b) to determine whether the rights and welfare of any such subjects will be adequately protected; and (c) to determine whether legally effective informed consent will be obtained by adequate and appropriate methods.[39] That there were three co-equal requirements of review suggests that the writers of the regulations believed that the right to consent as well as the other "rights and welfare" mentioned in clauses (b) and (c) were not derived from the notion of risk to the subject. If they were, it would be more appropriate to say that the review committee must see that the risks to the subject *including violations of rights* are so outweighed. . . . The 1974 DHEW regulations followed traditional theories of rights in American political philosophy by recognizing that rights of individuals including the right to consent are independent of consideration of risks.

Yet if that is so, it is paradoxical that (b) and (c), that is, the protection of rights including the right to consent, were to be assured by review only in cases where the subject was at risk. Logically it would make sense to require that a determination of risks was sufficiently outweighed by potential benefits only in cases where subjects are at risk, but it is inconsistent to require that the rights of the subject are to be protected only in cases where the subject is at risk.

By contrast the DHHS regulations published in 1981 require review of all research involving human subjects. There is no limitation to research involving risk. However, certain research is exempt from the regulations, and, once again, it is primarily research that would normally be thought of as involving very low or no risk to the subjects. For example, research is exempt if it is conducted on existing medical records and the information is recorded by the investigator in such a manner that subjects cannot be identified.[40] These exemptions still ignore the fact that a subject might object to having the investigator see the record (especially if the investigator were known to the subject). They also ignore the possibility that the subject might object to the purpose of the study. If records were used, for example, some subjects might object even if they are not placed at risk of harm. Subject autonomy is in jeopardy even if subject welfare is not. Patients are hardly partners in the process if they do not even know they are participating.

If it is correct that the principle of autonomy is the proper foundation of a theory of informed consent and that rights of subjects exist independent of consideration of risks and benefit, then there seems to be only one possible explanation of the subordination of the determination of protection of subject rights to the determination that the subject is at risk. To make this clear let me suggest two forms of the notion of self-determination that might be viewed as a basis for informed consent.

The first I would call the weak theory of self-determination. According to this view an individual has the right to self-determination regarding invasion of his body or his privacy only when exercising that self-determination will materially affect his welfare. In this case an individual's right to self-determination is limited to the area of risk-taking. Alternatively, we can consider a "full" or "strong" theory of self-determination. If individuals are always to be treated as ends and never as means, those individuals are the possessors of autonomy in all areas of life, not simply in cases when material risks and benefits are at stake. In fact at least within limits we shall consider below, they possess the right to self-determination to make choices that are contrary to their own interests. Put in these terms it seems most implausible that the rights of life, liberty, and the pursuit of happiness would carry the proviso "only in circumstances when risks and benefits are involved." Many of the cases where one exercises the right to self-determination are cases in which risks of harms and benefits as we normally think of them are not at stake. The constitutional rights to liberty and privacy are not so limited that they only apply in cases where a committee has determined that the subject is at risk.

If one examines the standard lists of basic elements of informed consent, one discovers that some of the items included are not directly linked to the subject's calculation of risks and benefits. For instance, suppose human blood were needed to develop a test for sickle cell anemia and trait in fetuses. Blood samples are to be obtained from adults with and without sickle cell disease or trait for purposes of developing the test. The eventual objective of the research is to develop the diagnosis in time so that all fetuses with disease or trait could be aborted, thus improving the gene pool. If the blood were obtained as remaindered blood from routine diagnostic work, it is difficult to conceive of any risk to subjects in having it used in the study. They will never be at risk to be aborted as a fetus and, if they already have reason to believe they and their spouse do not have the disease or carrier status, their offspring could not even be affected in any direct manner.[41] Yet it seems that some people might object to the purposes of this research. It will eventually lead to aborting black fetuses. Still more might object to having their blood used for this study without their consent. That presumably is why the first basic element of informed consent includes a fair explanation of the *purposes* of the research.

A second example of a piece of research where no plausible risk to the subject is at stake and yet subjects might plausibly want the opportunity to consent to the research involves a study using human placentas for basic physiological study. Placentas routinely discarded in the delivery room would be salvaged for research purposes. It could plausibly be argued that the women from whom the placentas were taken were not at risk from the study. They were not being asked to modify the delivery procedure at all. Yet it seems plausible that many women would want to be told that the placenta was to be used in this manner. Some may object; others would gladly consent—if they are given the opportunity.

A third example is studies of patient compliance with medical instructions mentioned by Levine.[42] Even if one had no reason to fear direct risk of ridicule, one might plausibly object to the concept of "compliance" on the grounds such research is often built on the unstated hypothesis that patients are wrong in their judgment not to follow medical advice (or "doctor's orders"). If one believed that such patient judgments were often rational, given the value system and world view of the patient, but also that those studying "compliance" did not share that belief, then one might want to refuse to participate in such compliance studies on the grounds that they were misguided, had the potential of leading to erroneous conclusions, and, if nothing more, were paternalistic in their conception. Such a patient might reasonably want the opportunity to consent to participate in such studies because he or she objects to the purpose of the study rather than the risks.

Even the use of autopsy material and severed organs and limbs for research raises questions which certain individuals would find potentially meaningful or useful. For instance, Orthodox Jews might object on theological grounds to autopsy and subsequent research use unless they were directly linked to the saving of a particular life.[43] Objections to the purpose of the research as well as idiosyncratic objections based on unique systems of belief and value can be made independent of risk/benefit considerations. The point is a logical one: If the right of self-determination is the proper basis of the consent, it is illogical to make the exercise of that right dependent upon the subject's being at risk.

II. THE STANDARD OF REASONABLY INFORMED CONSENT

If the proper theoretical foundation for informed consent is the principle of self-determination or autonomy, this ought to have implications for our understanding of informed consent in various research settings. Before looking at those implications for specific settings, I want to connect this self-determination theory to an issue that has received much attention recently in the legal literature: the problem of determining the standard to be used in deciding how much information ought to be transmitted for a consent to be informed.

Before looking at some plausible alternative answers it is necessary to put aside one red herring, the standard of "fully informed and free consent." Researchers sometimes argue that it is impossible to give the subject enough information for consent to be "fully" informed.[44] To do so would require an infinite amount of information—or at least a full medical education. Since consent cannot be fully informed, they argue, the physician should select particularly important items to transmit, but not strive for an impossible standard.

I claim this is a red herring because no one, or at least no one who has carefully thought about it, really demands "fully" informed consent. It is not only impossible, but would be terribly tedious. It is more plausible to require that all potentially useful or meaningful information be transmitted. (I say meaningful as well as useful since, as in the case of the placentas, some information might be seen as meaningful even if no concrete use can be made of it.)

We are still left with the question of how much information ought to be transmitted if the standard is that which is potentially useful or meaningful. Most believe that the traditional standard was some variant on the standard of the profession: what the reasonable physician would have disclosed under the circumstances.[45] The court case which is often cited is Natanson v. Kline, especially the qualification that:

> The duty of the physician to disclose, however, is limited to those disclosures which a reasonable medical practitioner would make under the same or similar circumstances. How the physician may best discharge his obligation to the patient in this difficult situation involves primarily a question of medical judgment . . . the physician's choice of plausible courses should not be called into the question if it appears, all circumstances considered, that the physician was motivated only by the patient's best therapeutic interests and he proceeded as competent medical men would have done in similar circumstances.[46]

The standard of the profession has been challenged widely in court cases in ten states[47] and in many articles in legal journals.[48] This legal development I take to be the most exciting theoretical conceptual shift in the ethical and legal dimensions of medicine in the twentieth century.

From Justice Schroeder's opinion in Natanson v. Kline it appears that patient benefit is an underlying concern for setting the standard of how much information is to be transmitted. The physician is to be motivated only by the patient's best therapeutic interests. Even if one assumes that patient benefit is the primary foundation of informed consent—an assumption that we have challenged and that would rule out all non-therapeutic experiments—it would still be necessary to make further assumptions in order for the standard of the profession to be used in determining how much information must be transmitted. It would be necessary to assume that the physician or physician/researcher was the proper person to determine what is in the patient's best interest.

This presumption appears to rest on an old model of medical decision making, one that sees medical choices as essentially technical matters based on the scientific skills of the physician. If we can presume that the values underlying the decision are agreed upon and the only question is which medical practices would promote the desired end, then those with technical competency would appropriately be able to decide what would be in the patient's interest.

If consent for experiments were based upon either subject benefit or broader societal benefit and we can assume there is some one more expert than the subject himself in deciding what is beneficial, then it would be plausible to limit the information transmitted to those items which the expert considered necessary in deciding what would be beneficial. Thus, apparently beginning from a patient-benefitting motive, Garnham proposes substitution of a physician's informed judgment for that of the patient's.[49]

Even if this were the theoretical underpinning of the consent, however, it is unlikely that the medical professional would be the appropriate expert at least unless he or she had sufficient psychological skills to decide what would benefit and what would harm. In cases of consent for experimentation, the subject-benefitting consideration, which might require getting consent or place limits on getting that consent, is primarily the psychological benefits to the patient/subject. If the patient/subject would be distressed at not knowing what was being done, then consent should be obtained. If the patient/subject would be distressed at hearing the details of the research or its purposes, then it should not be—according to this theory. But it would normally be psychological experts who could most appropriately make that judgment. If, on the other hand, consent is rooted in a *bonum commune* defense, then the appropriate expert would be someone such as a sociologist skilled at judging community sentiment about the research enterprise. In neither case would the (non-psychiatrist) physician have the *relevant* skills.

It seems clear, however, especially in cases when a decision must be made between using a conservative approach with an established therapy and a more innovative course with an experimental therapy, that the decision of which course is preferable depends on matters other than technical medical knowledge. Such a choice will be made on the basis of personal values and beliefs that are quite independent of medicine. Thus, such a decision is not the proper responsibility of the physician; rather, it is best left to the patient.

If the theory behind informed consent is the individual's right to autonomy or self-determination, however, then the appropriate standard for how much information should be transmitted should not be related to any professional skills. The standard ought to be the amount of information necessary for the subject to exercise self-determination, that is the amount of information the subject would find useful or meaningful, independent of whether the researcher or the research community would find that information useful or meaningful.[50] If the objective of the consent is to promote self-determination, then it is the subject population itself that must provide the standard for determining how much information is to be transmitted in order to exercise self-determination.

Earlier I said, with regard to the Natanson v. Kline case, that most *believe* that this case puts forward the traditional standard of the profession. In fact a close reading of it reveals it is much closer to the reasonable-person standard than most realize. In the earlier quotation a key phrase was omitted, one which is often overlooked. It says the standard of the profession is to be used in judging the adequacy of information "so long as the disclosure is sufficient to assure an informed consent." The fact that the patient-benefitting criterion and the standard of the profession are specifically qualified in this way suggests that Judge Schroeder must have had something more in mind.

This shift to lay standards—determining what the reasonable person would want to know before consenting to research or therapy—is now becoming the basis for judging whether a consent is informed. The "reasonable man" (or "reasonable person") standard is now explicit in court cases in many jurisdictions beginning with Berkey v. Anderson in California in 1969 in which it was argued that:

> We cannot agree that the matter of informed consent must be determined on the basis of medical testimony any more than that expert testimony of the standard practice is determinative in any other case involving a fiduciary relationship. We agree with appellant that a physician's duty to disclose is not governed by the standard practice of the physicians' community, but is a duty imposed by law which governs his conduct in the same manner as others in a similar fiduciary relationship. To hold otherwise would permit the medical profession to determine its own responsibilities. . . .[51]

There are radical implications for local experimentation committees of the reasonable-person standard for determining how much information is necessary for consent to be informed. I have elsewhere done a study of those implications.[52] Here I shall only summarize the conclusions.

One task of such committees is to determine if legally effective informed consent will be obtained. If, however, self-determination is the foundation for making that decision and therefore the reasonable layperson's judgment is necessary for deciding how much information that is, then a committee that is skewed in its composition away from that representative reasonable layperson will not be capable of deciding whether the consent proposed is adequate. If committees include research scientists in greater proportion than in the general public and those research scientists predictably give atypical answers to such questions as whether they would want to know certain information and whether the risk is "worth it" given the potential benefits of the knowledge, then such committees will give predictably unreliable answers to such questions. It is not just that the committee must include some lay representation. Rather in order to carry out adequately this one particular function of deciding what the reasonable layperson would want to know, the committee must be made up entirely of laypeople (or, alternatively, composed in such a way that special professional biases are neutralized). Of course, for other functions requiring technical expertise, such as establishing the risks, professional skills are needed. This remains a fundamental dilemma. One solution would be to have an all-lay committee with professionals used in a strictly technical advisory capacity. Another is to use lay "surrogates" to inform a professional committee of what laypeople would want to be told. The capacity of laypeople to make such judgments and the fact that those judgments differ from professionally staffed IRBs is documented by Norman Fost's study of a "surrogate system" for informed consent.[53] Fost asked parents who had recently given birth to a normal child to pretend they were to be participants in a study in which umbilical artery catheterization was to be performed on their newborn. He did this to suggest a model that might be used in the informed consent process. A similar strategy was tested by Richard Winer and several others including me as a way of measuring what persons in situations similar to potential subjects would want to be told in a consent process. The Winer study is presented for the first time in chapter 12 of this volume. The technique of using surrogates is an alternative to using an all-lay committee to determine what reasonable laypersons in the subject's position would want to be told.

Even if those with special medical skills and the unique value commitments that accompany those skills are limited to the role of technical advisors to an all-lay committee, there is reason to doubt that it is even theoretically possible, much less practical, to transmit information to the committee in a "neutral" manner. Perhaps we should consider shifting to the advocacy system for such review of protocols. Under such a system, technical staff selected purposely because of their inclination for and against the research enterprise would be charged with the tasks of presenting the best cases for and against the protocol under consideration. The lay committee members, having heard the cases, would, after an opportunity to request further information and explanation, exercise their judgments as reasonable people about the adequacy of the consent (and presumably also about whether the risk to the subject was justified by the potential benefit to subject and/or others).

There is one additional problem with the use of the reasonable-person standard for assuring that subjects will receive the information they consider useful or meaningful. What of the subject who is "unreasonable" in the technical sense the term "reasonable" is used in the law? What of the subject who desires more or less information than the reasonable person? If the goal is providing enough information for adequate self-determination, surely the reasonable-person standard is not adequate for such subjects. If there is any reason to believe that the particular patient or subject wants more information than the reasonable citizen, then the patient or subject's own standard of certainty must apply. This is sometimes referred to as the "subjective standard." If a subject communicates to researchers that he wants more information of a particular sort than the reasonable person would, there is an obligation of the researcher to give that additional information if the subject is to continue to be part of the experiment.[54] At least for non-therapeutic experiments, it ought to be sufficient for the researcher to drop such a subject from the research. For potentially therapeutic experiments the abandonment of the patient/subject by the physician/researcher when he or she has a treatment potentially beneficial to the patient/subject would raise the same problems of any physician abandonment. The obligation to give ample notice and reference to another physician willing to provide the treatment might be required—at least within the limits of reasonableness. That few other physicians may be capable of giving the experimental treatment makes the case more difficult than the normal therapeutic situation.

An even more difficult problem would be the case of the patient/subject who communicates that he or she wants less information than the reasonable person. Since I am contending that the principle of self-determination is the one that ought to be used in requiring informed consent, it might be possible to argue that the patient/subject should have the right to determine that there is some information he or she would rather not have. That, of course, does not make the patient/subject's request for less information an ethical request. If the human is ethically responsible for decisions about his or her own medical future, it can be seriously questioned at the ethical level whether one is justified in waiving information necessary to make a consent informed. Nevertheless, since the physician's role is not one of forcing ethical behavior on patients against their will, in cases of routine patient care such a waiver might be taken as sufficient to relieve the physician of an obligation to disclose.

In the case of experimentation, however, it cannot necessarily be concluded that a physician is justified in keeping a subject in a study when that subject has waived the right to the information necessary to make an informed decision about participation. The researcher has an option other than imposing information on the subject against his or her explicit instructions. It is an option that permits the investigator to be true to the obligation to get an adequately informed consent without imposing significant risks on subjects. While withdrawing from a patient-physician relationship in routine clinical medicine would impose a risk on a patient, by definition it would not in research. Research is conducted ethically either in cases where no therapy is involved or in cases where the alternatives are considered to have similar benefit-harm ratios. In such cases the investigator can turn to other subjects who are willing to receive the information necessary to make an informed choice. He can do so without compromising his own duty to inform and without imposing risks on the subject. That would seem to be the preferable course.

If the standard for an adequately informed consent is the standard of the reasonable person (modified in cases when there is evidence the subject differs from that standard), we are still left with the question of substance: What information must be transmitted? The exact content must be determined by reasonable representatives of the public on a case by case basis. Some basic elements of informed consent, however, spell out the kinds of information necessary. In addition to the elements currently included in DHHS guidelines,[55] there are some additional elements I believe a reasonable person would want to know before giving an adequately informed consent.[56] These include:

1. A specific disclosure of the presence of a control group within the research design.[57]
2. A statement of the "inconveniences" as well as the risks and discomforts.[58]
3. Names of review and patient-protection agents including the person in the institution and the person at the federal level who should be contacted if the subject has further questions about the experiment.
4. A statement of the rights of the subject. This should include not only the presently required statement of the right to withdraw without prejudice, but the right to access to the alternative treatments, mention of which is not presently required.
5. Explanation of who, if anyone, will be responsible for harms done to the subject. This should include an explanation of who, if anyone, will be responsible for both anticipated harms the risk of which was included in the consent, and negligent and non-negligent but unanticipated harms.
6. An explanation of the right, if any, to continue receiving treatment found helpful to patient/subject.

There are new elements that are necessary for a consent to be adequately informed, and should be added to those currently in the list of elements in the DHHS guidelines.[59] Many of the elements proposed by Robert J. Levine[60] should be included such as the requirement that there should be a clear invitation rather than a request or demand, that the subject be informed why he has been asked to participate in the study, and that there be a suggestion to the prospective subject that he or she might wish to discuss the proposed research with another before consenting. Levine's final element—consent to non-disclosure—does not specify the limits of the non-disclosure and thus is not justified though an amended form of it (which set limits to non-disclosure) may be. These limits are discussed below when considering research which could be destroyed if informed consent were obtained.

Levine's skepticism with the "short form" of the written consent document is well-founded.[61] The use of a short written form, which has the subject affirm that items have been explained orally, serves no useful purpose, especially since a written version must be on file with the IRB. In some cases it leads to suspicion about what is actually communicated, not necessarily because the researcher is not trusted, but because staff actually obtaining the consent may accidentally omit certain items. Levine's doubts about general-consent forms for categorically related research are also valid. They also fail to provide evidence of the actual consent should litigation arise. Both short forms and general-consent forms should be excluded as not assuring legally effective consent; I would thus favor deletion of paragraph 46.10(b) from the May 30, 1974, version of the DHEW policy.

Finally, there is one procedural problem in the mechanism of getting consent which I think needs correction. Whether a regular or a short written form is used, it seems to be too much to ask of a researcher that he negotiate the consent with the subject himself. The commitment of the researcher to the worthiness of the project and the justification of the risk on grounds of benefit to the subject and/or others are, or ought to be, very high—or he ought not to undertake the project in the first place. The conflict of interest is too great for a normal person to bear.[62] I would favor the use of those with no direct involvement in the protocol to negotiate the consent with the potential subject. (An alternative might be the negotiation first with the one hired as an advocate for the opposition to the subject's participation, then with the researcher.)

III. THE IMPLICATIONS OF THE SELF-DETERMINATION THEORY OF CONSENT

What then are the implications of the self-determination theory of informed consent for subjects in different research settings? The implications will depend upon the setting. In this final section I shall discuss, first, subjects which I (would) call *Group I subjects*, competent, non-institutionalized adult subjects receiving private medical care. Then I will turn to the implications of the self-determination principle for *Group II subjects*, subjects whose capacity to consent is compromised in some way.

A.   GROUP I SUBJECTS

The theory that consent for participation in research is rooted in the principle of autonomy has implications first for those subjects ideally placed to give consent that is relatively free and informed. If we limit ourselves to Group I subjects for non-therapeutic research (i.e., subjects who are mentally competent, non-institutionalized adults who receive health care through private channels), we have probably limited ourselves to the group most capable of exercising self-determination. Some implications are apparent even for this group.

First, if self-determination is the objective, then consent is necessary for research independent of the risk involved. Second, recognizing that self-determination is always a relative phenomenon, determining how much information will be necessary for autonomous decision making insofar as the goal is promoting self-determination will have to be based on standards as close as possible to the subject's own. Normally this will mean the consensus of reasonable laypersons, but modified as necessary to bring the standard in line with ways in which the subject may be known to differ from the reasonable layperson.

Third, there may be limits to that to which the layperson may acceptably consent. This is a problem that I have not taken up because it takes us beyond the nature and definition of informed consent. Even though informed consent may be rooted in a principle of autonomy, there may be other constraints on participation in research beyond the right to self-determination. In a society as thoroughly committed to individual liberty as ours is, discretion may be very broad, but there may nevertheless be limits.

Even the arch defender of liberty John Stuart Mill recognized at least two limits to liberty. The first limit is harm to others.[63] It is unlikely that experiments could be banned when subjects give free and informed consent on the grounds that they would do harm to others, but such objections are conceivable, for instance, in a viral transduction experiment performed to manipulate the human genetic code where both researcher and subject are adequately informed and willingly agree to participate in the study.

Although it is not generally recognized, Mill also places a second limit on liberty: the limit of prohibiting surrender of one's own liberty.[64] Thus, Mill believes it could never be justified to sell oneself into slavery. It is possible that some free and informed consents by subjects of Group I would be seen even by Mill as surrendering too much liberty, for instance, volunteering to take great risk of death for marginally valuable results or volunteering for experimental brain manipulation. Such consents could be attacked as not truly free or not adequately informed, but the mandate of local review committees would permit such prohibitions even if the consent were considered free and informed. The committee must determine not only if there is informed consent, but independently, whether the risks to the subjects are adequately outweighed by the potential benefits to subject and/or others. If the right of self-determination for the competent, non-institutionalized adult is taken seriously, the instances when that right should be compromised on paternalistic grounds will be extremely limited if not non-existent. Occasionally, in an experiment that was analogous to selling oneself into slavery as in the Beaumont experiments, experimentation with free and informed consent might be rejected on the grounds that the subject's liberty cannot voluntarily be surrendered. For the most part, however, a prohibition of a person who has given informed consent from participating in an experiment would have to be based on the state's role as protector of the welfare of its citizens, and instances of this are rare indeed. There are limits to liberty in our society—until recently men could be drafted to risk life and limb—but in even those cases the conscription was done in the name of protecting liberty itself. Blocking of experiments in which there is free and informed consent solely on the independent grounds of paternalism is rarely, if ever, justified. On the contrary, prohibiting experiments on grounds of general welfare to society may be justified but only in the event that the liberty of society is seriously threatened.

B.   GROUP II SUBJECTS

Although I recognize the dangers of overgeneralization, I will call all groups of subjects where the capacity to consent is problematic Group II subjects. I treat them all as a single group because they all, in some way, are subjects whose autonomy is problematic. Generally, since we should not treat people as a means without their consent, we should conduct research on patients in this group only when research on Group I patients is impossible (and I mean impossible, not merely inconvenient). While therapeutic interventions, even non-standard interventions, may upon occasion be justified on grounds of the welfare of the patient, research itself is not justified on these grounds. For research, which necessarily includes elements of interventions for the purpose of gaining knowledge, consent of substantially autonomous persons must, at least when possible, be a prior condition in addition to beneficence. Only in cases when the class of Group II subjects as a whole could be benefitted, when it is reasonable to conclude that they would or should consent if they could, and when the benefit could not possibly be gained by studies on consenting subjects, should research on them be considered.

1.   Children

The clearest example of the impossibility to exercise self-determination is the very young child. In the small child, consent has a very limited applicability because self-determination is very limited. It is a mistake, for the most part, to speak of "proxy consent" for experiments in children. Rather what is at stake should be precisely clarified: Research without subject consent is justified, if at all, on some other grounds. For therapeutic research on young children we must fall back in part on a principle which we have seen is highly suspect: the principle of patient benefit. Therapeutic research, by definition, proposes experimental treatments about which there is no consensus as to the benefits. Therefore, it is never possible to justify such experiments solely on patient-benefit grounds. The justification must be supplemented with the requirement that we should at least insist that there is no significant unfavorable benefit/harm ratio. In addition, we might add a hypothetical variant of a consent requirement by insisting that it is reasonable to conclude that the subjects themselves would or should consent if only they were capable of understanding.

Parental "approval" or "selection"[65] of subjects for such therapeutic research is essential for two reasons: First, under the norm of patient benefit, parents in their guardian role are obligated to serve the best interests of their children. They are in the best position to protect their interests, to assure that patient welfare is not significantly jeopardized. Second, since in cases of therapeutic experiment there is no consensus about what would be in the child's best interest, parents are given very limited discretion to choose values upon which decisions may be made for their children. It is in this second role that parental approval takes on the aura of a consent. Parents in our society are given limited authority to exercise *their own* self-determination about the values of their offspring. They are permitted to select religious training, parochial education not valued by the majority, vegetarian or "organic" diet, and other values not generally shared by the ordinary person. In this one sense parental "consent" is the appropriate term. The willingness of courts to intervene if parental determination of values deviates very far from the social consensus is an indication of the limitation of parental consent; for instance, if Amish parents were to choose no school rather than, as in the case of parents choosing parochial education, a minority school.

One of the areas in which parents are permitted to exercise some discretion is in encouraging the child to make minor contributions to the general welfare or to the welfare of specific others. Parents may encourage the child to contribute a small portion of his allowance to the Red Cross; however, the limits of parental discretion are quite narrow. The child is not the property of the parent. Non-therapeutic research may be one area where parental self-determination is to be tolerated within these narrow limits.

One main line of opinion holds that no child or other non-consentable can ever be the subject of non-therapeutic research because he cannot consent, and a human should never be treated as a means rather than an end unless consent is obtained.[66] This, however, is a highly individualistic understanding of moral responsibility. If, in addition to being an end in himself with inalienable rights, the individual is seen as a member of a social community, then certain obligations to the common welfare may be presupposed even in cases where consent is not obtained. The dangers of balancing individual rights with obligations to serve the common welfare are great especially in cases where consent cannot be used as a mechanism to judiciously waive those rights. In very special cases, however, where no risk or minimal risk to the subject is envisioned and when information to be obtained from experiments on children would be of great value and can be obtained in no other way, there must be some contribution to the general welfare which can be expected *without consent.* Just as parents may reasonably conclude that up to some minimal level their children ought to share their toys or their food, so they may reasonably conclude that they ought to share in contributing to scientific research. While autonomy would still lead to acceptance of subject refusals in such cases, where the subject cannot refuse, parental permission should make participation acceptable. This is not to say that social benefits can cancel individual rights, that patient benefit can be traded interchangeably for social benefit. It is rather to say that it is reasonable to treat the individual, non-consenting subject as a means to an end under very limited and circumscribed conditions.

Even if it is emphasized that this is not the same as making the utilitarian trade-off, there are great dangers in such a proposal. For this reason, parental approval of non-therapeutic research in such special cases should be required first, as the best check to make sure that individual rights are not unduly compromised and, second, to permit parental self-determination to be decisive in deciding whether their offspring will make a justifiable but non-consenting contribution to the general welfare.[67]

All of this is said with regard to consent and parental approval for very young children where no self-determination is possible. It seems to me to be valid also for older children. However, there are two special problems. For children old enough to communicate, assent is possible although that assent may be neither free nor informed. Since the child has nothing to gain, it seems reasonable that his uninformed refusal should nevertheless be determinative. In addition to free and informed parental approval and the constraints on that approval (for the reasons given above), uninformed assent of the child should also be required.

Normally this argument about the assent of incompetent subjects is limited to research involving procedures unrelated to therapy. I have increasing doubt that such a limitation is justified. Research is, as we have seen, by its very nature not for the benefit of subjects. It may be conducted on procedures that are for the benefit of subjects. In some cases it is unclear whether a standard or an innovative treatment is preferable. In those cases randomization is justified if the competent subject consents. If he or she refuses, the randomization is forbidden. I see no reason to limit the assent requirement to competents. If relative indifference between the two treatment alternatives is a prerequisite for justifiable randomization and the incompetent patient rejects one of the treatments for some reason, no matter how irrational, little would be lost by giving the patient the preferred alternative. The assent of the incompetent would appear to be a requirement even for so-called therapeutic experiments.

Finally for older youth, some real self-determination may be possible.[68] If a youth could exercise self-determination, I see no reason why that should not take precedence over parental judgment. The problem, of course, is determining that the youth's judgment is free and informed. Two solutions seem possible: generally lowering the age of majority so that youth can consent on their own or making such judgments on a case-by-case basis. For some medical *treatments* lowering the age of consent for the particular treatment (such as venereal disease and birth-control services) may be justified. In general, however, I think it is wiser to keep the age of consent for medical treatment high—at least 18. To adopt a general lower age for consent for medical treatment might mean substituting the persuasion of the medical profession or others with influence for the authority of the parent. For research and for treatments not covered by a specific statute lowering the age for consent, case-by-case adjudication of the judgment of the youth disagreeing with parental judgment seems appropriate.

2. *Formerly Competent Adults*

Formerly competent adults—mental patients, the comatose, and the senile—are, for purposes of consent, very similar to children in that they lack the capacity to exercise self-determination. They differ, however, in several important regards. They were formerly competent; at one time in the past they could exercise self-determination. In some instances formerly competent individuals may have expressed disapproval of experimental cancer treatments or expressed a desire to contribute to scientific knowledge of their particular disease. While in young children the parental judgment about what is in the child's interest would be taken as decisive within limits, in the case of the formerly competent adult the situation is more complex. There is currently great debate about whether statements about medical treatments written while competent ought to remain valid when one is no longer competent.[69] Some argue that if the incompetent patient were able to have an opinion now when incompetent, his opinion would have changed, that it is impossible for the healthy individual to anticipate the experience of terminal illness or chronic mental incapacity. On the other hand, what judgment could be more reliable about the wishes of the now incompetent one than the wishes of that person expressed while competent? I take it to be an assault on the principle of autonomy to hold that statements made while competent are unacceptable expressions of the best estimate of what one would want when and if incompetent.

There is a second problem with incompetents lacking in the case of children. While statute normally specifies when a child is a minor incapable of giving consent for medical treatment and research, the definition of incompetency in adults is much more tenuous. The circle defining those who are incompetent is shrinking rapidly. Many patients, including some committed to mental institutions, who were formerly considered incompetent to accept or refuse medical treatments are now being permitted to do so.

An institutionalized woman in depression was permitted to refuse the continuation of electroshock therapy.[70] A 60-year-old committed schizophrenic was permitted to refuse a breast biopsy for diagnosis of a possible malignancy on the grounds that she might die, that it would interrupt her movie career, and prohibit her from having further children.[71] In New York, the state health code explicitly specifies that mental patients are permitted to refuse experimental treatments.[72] Experiments on mental patients and other formerly competent subjects should be under the same restrictions as for youth, subject to wishes expressed while competent, except in rare cases where they might be justified when the knowledge sought cannot be gained in any other manner, when there is no risk or minimal risk, when there is informed approval by a guardian, and when there is uninformed pro forma assent by the subject, when possible. Guardian approval or judicial determination that the patient is exercising adequate self-determination ought to be required. Expressions made while competent, however, should be taken as evidence of the patient/subject's wishes.

3. *Prisoners*

Although prisoners are frequently grouped with children and mental patients as difficult cases when discussing consent, the problems created in the case of prisoners are radically different. It is frequently noted that prisoners may not be free psychologically because of the coercive nature of the choices offered in the prison setting. It seems that the only solution to the constraint on the prisoner's exercising self-determination is the restructuring of the institution so that the choice to participate in experiments is more on a par with other options. This might require increasing income opportunities from other forms of prison employment. The only proposal that I find plausible within the present prison structure is that those wanting to do prison research pay to the prisoners—as a group—fees comparable to what it would cost to obtain subjects outside of prison while the individual subject would receive an amount determined to be proportionate to other income-producing opportunities considering risk and time involved. The difference could then be used by the prison population for educational or recreational purposes of their own choosing.[73]

The larger problem for consent for prison research from the perspective of an autonomy-based theory of consent seems to be in a different area. In contrast with children, the senile, and the mentally incompetent, there is no reason to presume that prisoners lack the capacity for self-determination. If self-determination is a fundamental right in our society, then we should be very cautious in infringing upon that right even in the name of protecting the individual's welfare. While prisoners do not lack the capacity to consent, a social judgment has been made that their right to self-determination should be greatly constrained. Depending upon one's theory of imprisonment, infringing upon self-determination is thought justified either for protection of the public interest, for rehabilitation, or for punishment for previous wrongs done. Thus the prisoner's general presumptive right to self-determination has been overridden.

The implication for the prisoner consent depends upon the theory of imprisonment. If the sole purpose of imprisonment is to protect the public—

to get the criminal off the streets—then it is hard to see why the prisoner's right to consent to research should in any way be compromised in principle. For rehabilitation exercise of the right ought to be encouraged. If, however, retribution is the basis of the imprisonment, conceivably that right could be limited. If one of the functions of prison research is to give the prisoner an opportunity to make amends for previous wrong to society and to regain his sense of personal worth, then some might argue that such a "privilege" should not be given. That may be the view of the American Medical Association in their statement in 1952 in which they state:

> Whereas, some of the inmates who have participated have not only received citations, but have in some instances been granted parole much sooner than would otherwise have occurred, including several individuals convicted of murder and sentenced to life imprisonment. . . . Resolved, that the House of Delegates of the American Medical Association express its disapproval of the participation in scientific experiments of persons convicted of murder, rape, arson, kidnapping, treason, or other heinous crimes, and also urges that individuals who have lost their citizenship by due process of law be considered ineligible for meritorious or commendatory citation. . . .[74]

Regardless of whether human beings are imprisoned for purposes of protection or retribution, I cannot accept this argument for depriving them of self-determination in consenting to experimentation. While some constraints on self-determination may be necessary, those constraints must be carefully circumscribed. There can be no general loss of basic human rights. Until recently being a prisoner brought what was called "civil death," the loss of all rights. That radical infringement of rights has been abandoned, however, in favor of a much more limited deprivation of rights. Self-determination in choices about medical treatment—including experimental treatment—and about making humanitarian acts ought not to be limited any more than it would be for other competent adults. If constraints are necessary because prisoner consent is feared to be de facto coerced—even when the economic incentive is removed—that is a failure of the system, which ought not to be attributed to any deprivation of the prisoner's right to self-determination in this area. It is particularly serious if prisoners are deprived of their right to potentially therapeutic experimental treatments for this reason.

4. Clinic Patients

Like prisoners, clinic patients do not in principle lack the capacity to consent, but may be coerced into consenting because of serious constraints on their options for receiving health care. Clinic patients—patients whose opportunities for self-determination may be limited although their capacity should not be—should be treated as Group II subjects just as are children, the mentally incompetent, and prisoners. However, since they do not lack the capacity to consent and their rights might be especially jeopardized if they were deprived of any opportunity to participate in research, I reject what at first seems plausible: banning of all research on clinic patients. Rather, they should be treated like other Group II subjects. In cases where the study cannot be done on Group I patients and where it is reasonable to conclude that the subjects would be willing to participate, they should be permitted to do so with their consent no matter how compromised. This applies especially to studies of improving the quality of clinic care. In fact, there may be some studies where it is overwhelmingly likely that subjects would benefit from participation. A randomized comparison of two high-level health insurance plans for the treatment of the poor would be an example. In such a case it surely makes no sense to argue that indigent clinic patients should be excluded just because they are in clinics where their autonomy is problematic. Although they could be at some hypothetical risk, the odds are overwhelming that either treatment arm will leave them better off than not being in the study. In such cases Group II patients should be permitted to participate.

5. *Subjects in Experiments When Consent Would Destroy the Research*
There is a final group of subjects whose right to self-determination is potentially compromised: subjects in experiments where getting informed consent would, due to the nature of the study, destroy the experiment. Research in psychology of perception where the design often requires deceiving the subject as to the purpose or procedures is an example of such an experiment. A study to test the difference in response between subjects receiving a placebo who are told there is a placebo in the design and those who are not told would be another.

First, it is important to distinguish between cases where consent would necessarily destroy the experiment and cases where it would simply make the experiment more inconvenient or difficult. Omitting consent merely for the convenience of the researcher is never tolerable. Further, in some cases it may be possible to be clever in designing protocols so that deception or other lack of informed consent would not be necessary. In some cases it is believed that consent would destroy the experiment without any adequate grounds for that belief. For instance, there is no evidence that demonstrates the harm to the experiment of telling subjects there is a placebo in the design of a drug study (never, of course, telling them whether they are receiving the placebo). It is possible that the reports from the subjects would be different—they may be more cautious in their reporting; but a convincing argument that the results obtained would be any less valuable has not yet emerged. In fact it could be argued that they would be more valuable, because the subjects would generally be on guard to make accurate reports. I believe that in all designs where a placebo is used, it should be a requirement of informed consent to state that there is a placebo in the design.

There will still, however, be research that cannot be done without deception of the subject. We have seen that 1974 DHEW requirements justify such omissions of informed consent.[75] We deduced that a principle of social benefits was necessary to omit consent in such cases. But not just any social benefit would justify the consent omission. That is clear in the DHEW guidelines. First, omissions were justified only when the consent would "surely invalidate objectives of considerable immediate importance," when "reasonable alternative means for attaining these objectives would be less advantageous for the subjects, and when the risk to any subject is minimal." Thus there is already a clear recognition that not just any social benefit is sufficient to waive the consent. In fact the requirement that reasonable alternative means for attaining these objectives would be less advantageous *for the subject* is a requirement which would possibly permit some therapeutic research deception, but would apparently prohibit all psychology studies using deception in normal subjects since the deception study is of no advantage to the subject whatsoever.

I think we both need to go further and have gone too far. I believe we may have gone too far if we rule out all deceptive experiments where only the good of society is at stake. At the same time we have not gone far enough in specifying what principles and what tests would justify waiving of the consent. Hans Jonas, in discussing non-disclosure in cases where disclosure would destroy the research, also takes a position that the subject's rights may be violated even though no harm is done: "Only supreme importance of the objective can exonerate it, without making it less of a transgression. The patient is definitely wronged even when not harmed."[76] Jonas seems to limit his argument to non-disclosure in cases of research on patients (which he calls "an outright betrayal of trust"). It seems, however, that the argument works equally for the non-patient subject.

Jonas also does not develop the argument about what would be sufficient to justify such a non-disclosure. It seems that the one instance where such non-disclosure would be justified, the one principle that might at times override the right to self-determination, must be rooted in the very concepts of self-determination and trust. If, and only if, there is good empirical evidence that the subject would not consider the deceptive withholding of information a violation of that trust, would I find the non-disclosure acceptable.[77] If, and only if, we can reasonably presume on the basis of specific empirical evidence that reasonable subjects would not have objected to participating in the experiment without their consent, would such omission be justified.[78]

This is an empirically testable proposition. For any experiment which would be destroyed if informed consent were obtained, researchers should be required to draw a sample from the subject population proposed in the protocol, to explain to these mock-subjects the research in mind including the benefits as well as the deception involved. Subjects should then be asked whether they would have objected to being an uninformed participant, had the research actually been done on them without their informed consent. If we can predict, based on that sample, using a reasonable confidence limit such as 95 percent that other subjects drawn from the same population would not object, then it seems to be a justifiable compromise of the real subjects' right to self-determination. It is indeed a compromise because even at that level of certainty we would sometimes be wrong in presuming the subject would approve of the deception. Nevertheless, this seems to be a reasonable compromise. If a lesser number of mock subjects, say only a majority, approved, that could hardly justify a presumption that all or virtually all the uninformed subjects would have approved of the deception.

C. THE NEED FOR SPECIAL REVIEW OF CONSENT IN GROUP II SUBJECTS

Because consent with all group II subjects is problematic, procedures are needed to assure that these subjects' right to self-determination is not violated—insofar as such a capacity exists. I favor a special second-level review of all research involving Group II subjects, a national board charged with reviewing all such protocols. There is good reason to suppose that Group II subjects, especially clinic patients, are now used as subjects because using them is the path of least resistance. Establishment of an additional level of review would provide additional incentive to use subjects whose capacity and/or opportunities to consent are not as problematic. There is sufficient evidence that local committees vary tremendously in their standards for approving consents, that such precaution seems necessary to protect the rights and welfare of these special groups of subjects whose ability to give effective informed consent is so problematic.

The August 23, 1974, draft of proposed regulations for protection of human subjects included an alternative to a national-level review of consent.[79] That draft proposed additional protection for research involving fetuses, abortuses, pregnant women, and in vitro fertilization. It was proposed that a local "consent committee" be established to monitor consents. The proposal could be expanded to cover all of what I have called Group II subjects. It has not been included in any future regulations.[80] The argument given against them—that it would cost too much in time, money, and social benefits—cannot be a definitive argument for jeopardizing the rights of subjects unless one is committed to a utilitarian calculus of social costs and benefits.[81] This argument, insofar as it is put forward by researchers, should at least not be taken as definitive by the representatives of the public since researchers are legitimately expected by society to have a unique value commitment to the social benefits of the research enterprise.

My own position, however, is not that the consent committees would impede social progress; I am not convinced that they would stand in the way of well-designed and executed research. Rather I am concerned that a second group completely independent of the special characteristics institutionalized into the local IRB and exposed sufficiently to the special problems of consent in problematic cases be given an opportunity to review the quality of the consent as well as the judgment that the jeopardy to the subject's interests, rights, and welfare is justified by the potential benefit to the subject and/or others. This would be most effectively done by a national committee. This seems to me to be a compromise preferable to the well-articulated and often reasonable demands that research be banned entirely on children, prisoners, and other Group II subjects.

D.   PRINCIPLES BEYOND AUTONOMY

In principle I see one ground other than the principle of autonomy that would justify experiments on human subjects. This would apply to all experiments including experiments requiring non-disclosure. It is often held, I believe correctly, that humans have a *prima facie* obligation to promote justice independent of the consequences. This has led to an exciting contemporary debate about the meaning of justice, a debate taken up in detail in the next chapter. The theory developed by John Rawls[82] and the more egalitarian variants of that theory[83] would consider some practices fair and even right even though they might deprive individuals of their right to self-determination. The justification, however, is not in the production of good social consequences on balance, but in promoting justice. A theory of informed consent could be derived from this theoretical work that would provide a very limited basis for sacrificing the rights and interests of the individual for the benefit of certain others who are less well off (but not society in general).[84] It is to the principle of justice that we turn now.

CHAPTER FOUR

Justice and Research Design

Institutional Review Boards, the federally mandated review bodies charged at the local level with reviewing research protocols to assure that the rights and welfare of human subjects are protected, are beginning to be faced with a new kind of issue. Over the past decade they have become accustomed to assessing the potential benefits of the research and determining whether those benefits justify the risks to the subjects. These assessments are based on the principles of beneficence. They have also grown accustomed to determining that consent is adequately informed, that confidentiality is maintained, and that the other rights of the subject are protected. These judgments are based, at least in part, on the principle of autonomy. Recently, however, they have begun to address the question of equity or justice in the design of the research and selection of subjects.[1,2] A new principle, the principle of justice, must be added to the normative framework to deal with these issues.

The problem of justice arises, for example, when subjects are selected from especially deprived or vulnerable groups.[3] Should an institutional review board (IRB) require of investigators that protocols be designed to maximize the benefits to the subjects, even if such a design lowers the overall anticipated benefit to the society of the study? Should an IRB permit researchers wanting to study blood of subjects with a history of hepatitis to obtain blood samples from adolescents in a juvenile detention center, where many youths have such histories? The samples could be obtained from the general population, but with greater difficulty. Is it acceptable to use seriously ill patients in randomized clinical trials when they might prefer a non-randomized design?

At issue is the ethical legitimacy of targeting the recruitment of research subjects from a group that might be presumed among the least well-off in the community and of the design of the research to benefit such groups. The population of the juvenile detention center might well constitute the epitome of a deprived minority group: young, black and Hispanic, educationally and economically disadvantaged, lacking in sophistication about how to "work" the social system, and having no alternatives for obtaining health care. At issue is whether it is *fair*, whether it is *just*, to add to these youths' burdens the additional burden of serving as a research subject. Recently, some have begun to insist that morality requires recruiting the subjects from the general population rather than concentrating on an already disadvantaged group or, if recruitment of least well-off groups is necessary due to the nature of the study, designing the study to maximize benefit to the subjects even if it means compromising the net benefits that would result to society in general.

I. THEORIES OF JUSTICE IN HUMAN-SUBJECTS RESEARCH

A. THE BELMONT PRINCIPLES

For help in understanding the arguments the IRBs must consider, a review of the ethical principles put forth by the Belmont Report may be useful.[4] Three principles are articulated in the report, the same three principles presented in this and the two previous chapters. The first—respect for persons—contains within it the principle of autonomy, the subject of the preceding chapter. It may help us understand the reservations of those who have doubts about the use of disadvantaged subjects. Since autonomy is a central element of the notion of respect for persons, one might argue that constrained residents, like those of the juvenile detention center or the terminally ill, might not be able to exercise a truly free choice about participation in the protocol the way members of the general population might. While this might account for some of the resistance, clearly free choice is not the core of the argument over the use of vulnerable groups. Elaborate precautions might be included in the protocol to ensure that no resident of the juvenile detention center or terminally ill patient would be forced or coerced to participate, that there would be no way of linking participation to the availability of health-care services or to any other benefit, and that freedom of choice would be the maximum available within the confines of the institution. Still, the question remains of determining under what conditions it is fair to include disadvantaged groups as research subjects or to include them disproportionately.

The second principle of the Belmont Report—beneficence—is the principle I discussed in chapter 2. It provides little help in explaining resistance to the inclusion of disadvantaged groups. It is conceivable that long-term, subtle harms to the subjects themselves, or to others, might come as a result

of using these subjects in the research. If so, that would provide a bene-
ficence-based argument for shifting to the general population. However, the
benefits of using these particular disadvantaged populations and the disutilities of the alternative are overwhelming. Recruitment of a sizable group
of adolescent hepatitis victims from the general population, for example,
would require either an enormous random sample or recruitment by advertising or referral, which might bias the sample unacceptably. In the case of
testing a drug on a terminally ill patient, for example, a cancer patient, it
makes no sense at all, after phase one trials, to test the experimental drug on
other groups of patients. It is precisely because they are so ill that they are
chosen for the research. The consideration of beneficence seems to favor
heavily the proposed use of special populations. Again, this principle does
little to explain the heated debate over the obligation of researchers to select
and to use subjects equitably.

The Belmont Report makes clear that for research to be ethically acceptable according to the National Commission, it must meet a third and
apparently independent criterion. It is not enough that benefits of the
protocol exceed its anticipated risks. That was never enough. Even the old
DHEW regulations required, independent of beneficence considerations,
that the rights of the subjects be protected and that consent be adequate.[5]
Even the old regulations acknowledged that ethics was not a matter of mere
consequences. Ethics was even then rightly thought to be a matter of rights
that could hold the tyranny of an exclusive focus on good consequences in
check.

The Belmont Report and the new DHHS regulations make clear that, in
addition to respect for persons (and the consent that autonomy requires), still
another criterion must be met over and above producing good consequences
on balance. The new regulations require an IRB to make sure that the
"selection of subjects is equitable."[6] In adding the new mandate to the IRB
the regulation writers have finally acknowledged what the National Commission knew before them and what moralists have known for millennia: one of
the essential principles of morality is the just (or equitable) distribution of
benefits and burdens within a population.

Aristotle, in the fifth chapter of his *Nicomachean Ethics*, introduces us
to the first problem in the discussion of the principles of justice: the term
itself is exceedingly ambiguous. On the one hand, Aristotle tells us, justice
can be used very broadly—what he calls "complete justice."[7] Used in this
way, it means "complete virtue or excellence," or perhaps complete right-
ness. It is a synonym for the right or the morally correct.

Moderns concerned about a theory of justice are not using the term this
way, however. They have in mind Aristotle's second sense—what he calls
"partial justice" or "fairness in distribution."[8] It is the ethical principle that
addresses the narrower problem of how benefits and burdens should be
spread around, of whether the easily accessible resident of the juvenile
detention center should bear the burden of being asked to be a research

subject or whether terminally ill patients should be randomized in a clinical trial.

Distributional questions like this are relatively new to medical ethics. The Hippocratic tradition with its hyperindividualism is silent on such questions. The Hippocratic oath tells us nothing about how physicians ought to distribute their time and talent. That is why the traditional Hippocratic ethics of the physician cannot be used in assessing research protocols. In the nineteenth century, when systematic, controlled research was done for the purpose of gaining knowledge and when public health became an established component of modern medicine, medicine became social. Questions of distribution could no longer be avoided. The twentieth century has resolved the problem by adding independent principles such as autonomy and justice to the older moral norm of beneficence.

Justice addresses the question of how burdens and benefits should be distributed if the result is to be a *fair* one. Those individuals working in a narrow field such as the ethics of medical research immediately face a conceptual problem: should a principle of justice directly address narrow questions such as how the benefits and burdens of participation in research should be distributed, without *first* determining the more general problem of how general welfare, happiness, or general resources should be distributed? It seems obvious that what we are most fundamentally interested in seeking is how the more general primary or basic goods should be distributed. Thus any theory that directly attacks the justice of subject selection will be suspect. A just method of subject selection is most cogently determined by applying the most cogent general theory of justice to the specific problem of selection. Thus we need to examine the leading competitors for a theory of justice.

B.   FOUR THEORIES OF JUSTICE

There are four leading views on the question of how benefits and burdens would be fairly distributed. The first two envision the answer to the distributive justice question to be derivable directly from the other two principles, autonomy and beneficence. One of these views, libertarianism, holds that the fair way to distribute is simply to respect the autonomy of persons and to let the goods and the harms fall where they may. The other view, utilitarianism, holds that beneficence should be maximized and that we should accept the distributional results. The other two views of justice do not derive a principle of justice from the principles of autonomy or beneficence. They are Rawls's theory of justice and the egalitarian theory. Each of these presumes the principle of justice is independent from the principles of autonomy and beneficence.

1. A Libertarian View of Justice

The first interpretation of justice is that people are treated fairly if their autonomy is respected. It attempts to reduce the question of justice to one of respect for persons or autonomy. It is a theory that originates from modern

Western liberal political philosophy and has its most respected recent incarnation in Robert Nozick's *Anarchy, State, and Utopia*. According to Nozick, one is entitled to what one possesses provided it was acquired justly: from appropriation of goods not previously possessed, by gift, or by exchange. The state's role is simply to protect against unjust transfer.[9] By this notion the IRB's role would be reduced to one of assuring that no one's liberty and bodily resources are appropriated without the free agreement of the subject. It takes the existing abilities, talents, power, and status of individuals as a given. If a group of subjects such as the residents of the juvenile detention center or the terminally ill have little power, few resources, and no alternatives, but bargain freely to participate in research, they have, by this conception, been treated fairly.

This, of course, is not really a theory of justice in the traditional sense at all, i.e., in the sense of providing an equitable pattern of distribution of the subjects of the research or of the burdens of participation in the research. Nozick defends this view, nevertheless, since he believes it is a mistake to regard distributive justice as unquestionably a matter of filling in the blanks "from each according to_____, to each according to_____." Thus he prefers the term "justice in holdings" to distributive justice since the latter *presumes* a redistribution ought to take place. If he were to fill in the blanks above, Nozick says justice in holdings requires "from each as they choose, to each as they are chosen." His theory regards autonomy and freedom as absolute vis-à-vis distributive justice as it is traditionally conceived.

The libertarian theory has been attacked on at least two grounds. First, it has been pointed out that in this day no one has obtained anything by appropriating it as a good not previously possessed and that goods are so fundamentally social that the individualism of the libertarians no longer has any meaning. The research enterprise itself—the knowledge used by the researchers as well as the social structure that makes money, authority, and the subjects available—is fundamentally communal.

Second, it is asked even if goods were privately possessed, why would mere possession—based on luck, God-given ability, power, or fate—make the resulting pattern a fair or just one? The libertarian principle might maximize liberty, but why would we expect it also to enhance justice in the distribution of resources? Only if justice can be reduced to respect for the autonomy of persons will the Nozickian libertarian principle of distribution be adequate for an IRB in deciding how subjects can fairly be recruited.

2. *A Utilitarian View of Justice*

A second interpretation of justice tries to reduce justice to the principle of beneficence rather than to that of autonomy or liberty. The utilitarians, such as John Stuart Mill in chapter 5 of his *Utilitarianism*, claim that an adequate account of a fair distribution is given by simply trying to maximize the total net good produced by choices.[10] Mill states, in other words, that the principle of justice is already included in the principle of utility. This is the favorite representation of the health planners and of many researchers. The goal is the greatest good for the greatest number in aggregate net benefits. Distribution is on the basis of social contribution rather than ability. The principle justifies so-called non-therapeutic research on human subjects, which would always be immoral from the more individualistic ethical principles benefitting the patient advocated in the Hippocratic tradition. The trouble is that the principle justifies too much. It justifies research on human subjects without their consent or even against their consent provided the good produced in aggregate by the research is large enough. The principle of beneficence standing by itself as a basis for selecting human subjects certainly justifies using groups of disadvantaged subjects. The trouble is it also would justify the medical experiments carried out by the Nazis if only the benefits from the studies had been great enough. The IRB's mandate to assure that subject selection is equitable cannot mean simply that the IRB must justify selecting groups of subjects who would be severely harmed by the research and who are already among the population's most disadvantaged—provided that more good *in aggregate* comes from this selection compared to any other possible course.

The utilitarian beneficence principle does not take into account the distributions of benefits and harms. It takes no account of the fact that some small group may be harmed enormously while another, larger group is benefitted. Morally it does matter who is harmed and who is helped. The libertarian interpretation at least recognizes this. Libertarians recognize some individual claims even if it does not maximize utility. There is no logical reason why we should be interested in the total aggregate good—at least not when we are worried primarily about what is fair.

3. *A Maximin Principle of Justice*

The two remaining interpretations of the principle of justice take justice seriously as a way of producing morally acceptable patterns of distribution. Both interpretations view justice as an independent moral principle thereby placing demands on an IRB that differ from those of respect for persons and of beneficence. One of these interpretations, often called the maximin theory, claims that the demand of justice is not to maximize aggregate net benefit (as the utilitarians would hold), but to institutionalize practices that maximize the position of the least well-off members of the society. The maximin interpretation, defended most articulately by John Rawls in his *A Theory of Justice*, is a major challenger of the alternative simpler theories.[11] The fair thing to do, according to Rawls, is to develop social institutions and practices so as to improve the lot of the most disadvantaged members of the group. One thus maximizes benefits but only to the extent that the group having the minimum benefits (hence, "maximin"). The interesting feature of this interpretation is that the maximin principle may actually result in a decrease in the aggregate amount of benefit for the society as a whole. In research medicine the IRB's strategy would have to be, first, to identify the least well-off group. That in itself is a complex task raising basic problems of Rawlsian theory which require further attention. It would then have to ask how the protocol could be structured so as to maximize benefit for that group. If the juvenile detention center residents seem to be a least well-off group (in comparison to other potential subject groups), the research design would have to maximize benefits and minimize burdens to them. It is, of course, a matter of empirical debate whether a group such as the detention center residents are a least well-off group. It can also be debated on empirical grounds whether these residents would be benefitted or harmed by participation in the study. If it was determined that they would benefit, then, insofar as justice is concerned, they should be singled out as subjects even if it were more efficient to use some other group. If it was determined that they would be burdened on balance, then, insofar as justice is concerned, they should be spared participation even if it were less utility maximizing to use some other group. Determining whether subjects are likely to be benefitted or burdened on balance is itself a complex problem.[12] Devices such as community consultation have been proposed to assist in that assessment.[13] The fact that it would be more difficult to conduct the study using other subjects would be included in a calculus of beneficence, but not in that of a maximin strategy, which considers equity of research subject selection.

If the strategy of maximizing the position of the subjects with the minimum benefits is adopted, IRBs have a new and major item on their agendas: A protocol may satisfy all of the requirements of the old regulations (that the rights of the subject be protected and that consent be adequate) and yet still not be just or fair. In adopting a maximin approach to the question of equity, IRBs would have to begin asking whether the protocol maximizes the position of the least well-off.

4. The Egalitarian Theory

There is a fourth alternative interpretation of the principle of justice that also takes into account how benefits and harms are distributed. It is even more radical in its implications than the Rawlsian maximin theory.[14, 15] Rawls is now being attacked from the left by those who claim that even focusing on the benefit to the least well-off group might lead to very unequal amounts of benefits for different members of the society. These critics defend an egalitarian interpretation of the principle of justice, holding that the goal is not really to maximize the position of the least well-off, but to get the distribution of benefits and burdens as equal as possible.

Consider the following problem: Should elites in a society be given priority when doses of a potentially lifesaving drug become available? According to the Rawlsian formula focusing on benefit to the least well-off, the elites should be given the special priority if (of course, only if) giving them that advantage will create benefits to the least well-off (because the recipients would survive to treat the least advantaged, do research important to the welfare of the least advantaged, etc.). Under this condition, granting priority to the elites would be justified; it would be fair or just.

Egalitarians reject this conclusion. They say that it may be the right thing to do—especially if the least well-off consent to giving up their claim on the drug. They say, however, it cannot be the fair or just way to distribute the chance to get the drug. The egalitarian's goal is provision of an opportunity for all to be equal to others in the net amount of benefits they receive.[16] According to egalitarians, giving special priority to an elite who already have far more than their share of the benefits of the society cannot possibly be fair.

Both the maximin theorists and the egalitarians base their theories of justice on need rather than ability (central to the libertarians) or social utility (decisive for the utilitarians). However, they interpret the need standard in very different ways. The maximin theorists let elites have far more than an equal share of the goods, provided this helps to meet the needs of the least well-off. The egalitarian pushes need toward producing an equality of outcome—or at least to an opportunity for equality of outcome. In practice, the two interpretations of the needs-based principle of justice will often have the same policy implications. In principle, however, they are different.

C. THE RELATION TO OTHER PRINCIPLES

If either the Rawlsian or the egalitarian interpretation of the principle of justice is correct, then the IRB must face the question of how the demands of justice relate to those of autonomy and beneficence. The demands of the three principles may come into conflict. What does the IRB do when they do?

The easiest answers to that question, like most easy answers, turn out almost certainly to be wrong. For example, we might try to rank them giving absolute priority to beneficence or to autonomy. Almost everyone who has tried that approach, however, has concluded it will not work. In fact, this result is apparent from our previous discussion of the libertarians who assume autonomy is of paramount importance and of the utilitarians who assume that utility is such. Neither the National Commission nor the DHHS regulations gave rank ordering of principles.[17, 18] To do so could lead, if utility were ranked first, for example, to the conclusion that an IRB could approve protocols on grounds of great benefit even though they grossly violated the autonomy of subjects or the requirements of justice in distribution.

Another possibility is to balance the three principles so that a great violation for any one principle could offset a lesser violation of the other principles. This approach is far more attractive. Many philosophers, such as W. D. Ross, have opted for this clumsy, yet intuitively plausible, resolution.[19] That would mean, for example, that egalitarians could say that giving elites priority for an experimental drug violated the demands of justice, but so promoted beneficence and, with the consent of the rest of society, respect for persons as well, that justice should be sacrificed in this case.

There is no evidence, however, that the National Commission or the writers of current regulations opt for this strategy. They simply require that all three principles be satisfied. That is a third possibility. At least in research medicine, where by definition one is not sure benefit will come from the intervention, IRBs should bend over backwards to make sure subjects are protected, refusing to approve protocols until all three principles of ethics are satisfied simultaneously. In the case of a detention center hepatitis study, that would mean that since the IRB is not sure that justice is satisfied, even if they were sure that beneficence and autonomy were satisfied, the protocol could not be accepted until the subject selection better met the criterion of equity.

There is one other option, however, which may be even more attractive. The balancing strategy may be combined with the rank ordering of principles. For example, it may be autonomy and justice are coequal first principles that in some cases simply have to be balanced against each other, but together they always take priority over the principle of beneficence. This is the strategy I have recently attempted to defend.[20] This would mean that an IRB should be willing to sacrifice net benefit from a protocol in order to make sure that persons' autonomy was respected and subjects were treated fairly.

II. IMPLICATIONS FOR RESEARCH

Regardless of which solution is chosen for the problem of relating the three principles of autonomy, beneficence, and justice, IRBs will have to wrestle with the implications of the principle of justice. Assuming that one of the independent interpretations of the principle of justice is the correct one, so that justice does not simply reduce to autonomy or beneficence—an assumption that seems rightly justified in the new regulations and the Belmont Report—IRBs will have to decide independently whether a protocol meets the demands of equity. What will that mean in practice?

A. SUBJECT SELECTION

The most obvious impact on the IRB is indicated by the protocols involving disadvantaged groups. IRBs will have to struggle with the question of whether subjects have been selected equitably. It is by now common among IRBs to recognize that protocols involving certain classes of subjects should be singled out as raising areas of special concern. Protocols involving children, the mentally incompetent, prisoners, and fetuses are examples. Some of the problems involve either the autonomy of the subjects or the ability to understand and consent. I think it is now clear that these "suspect class" protocols (involving what in chapter 3 were referred to as Class II subjects) are also singled out because they are likely to raise problems of justice in the distribution of burdens and benefits. I have proposed that research recruiting subjects from clinic or ward populations be added to the list so that protocols involving these groups of subjects will be singled out for particularly rigorous scrutiny as well.[21] The burden of proof should be on the researcher to defend the use of children or prisoners.

Of course, some uses of groups that are socio-economically least well-off may well be justified. The obvious case would be a study of a problem unique to such a group. Study of a health-care delivery system for indigents would be an example. Other justifications, however, will be much more problematic. Convenience of the researcher in recruiting subjects, for example, may well be an unacceptable defense of the use of a ghetto clinic population. Fortunately, the choice of ward or clinic populations or of other groups singularly disadvantaged will often raise problems of scientific validity as well as ethical difficulties; thus there are scientific as well as ethical reasons for an IRB to suspect such protocols. However, the suggestion of an ethical question alone should trigger concern.

If the principle of equity requires *prima facie* that burdens and benefits of research be distributed to serve the interest of least advantaged groups and if subjects in suspect classes are assumed to be at high risk for being among the least well-off in society, then these subjects can justifiably be singled out for research only in cases where it can be assumed they will benefit on balance from participating. Of course, often in research, especially in medical research, if such an assumption is warranted, the intervention under study is not really at the experimental stage. Randomization involving control and experimental groups cannot be justified if it can be assumed that an experimental or control group will benefit significantly more than other groups.

It seems obvious that in special circumstances, as in social-policy research, some intervention will be beneficial, but researchers want to study the alternative methods of intervening, to determine which method is most beneficial or most efficient.[22] Studies of income maintenance, for example, meet these conditions.[23] In such a study, for example, an investigator might want to study the differential effects of guaranteeing income for a group of the poor at two levels. It is reasonable to assume that either "treatment" would be beneficial (although even this could be disproved). The purpose of the study is to examine which of two apparently beneficial interventions produces the most benefit. Targeting such a study for the poor might satisfy the principle of equity. In more ordinary situations, however, there is some real doubt whether experimental or standard treatment is more beneficial. When one considers the burdens on the subject of the data collection, the general nuisance of participation, and the risk of possible unanticipated side effects as well, the conclusion could be drawn that participating in a study involves higher probability of burden than benefit. This is probably true even if one takes into account the psychological rewards of participation and the potential benefits of treatment. This modest net burden to subjects is usually justified by the combined benefits to subject and to society that are anticipated along with adequate consent. But, if the net burden can be distributed to someone not in a least well-off group, the principle of equity calls for such subject selection.

B. RESEARCH DESIGN

The implications of a commitment to the principle of justice for subject selection should by now be apparent. However, there are other implications such as research design. Consider a research project to be conducted with seriously, perhaps terminally, ill patients where the objective is to study the effect of certain innovations in treatment. Let us begin with the premise that there is good reason to assume that the patient sick enough to be receiving an innovative treatment is a member of a least well-off group. If, after making this assumption, we consider only cases of research involving these kinds of patients, the demands of justice have enormous implications for the IRB.

If justice requires arranging the practices of research in order to benefit the least well-off and if in the protocol the sick patient being studied is presumptively a member of the least well-off group, then the researcher, the funders, the supervising institution, the society, and the IRB must adopt a radical new way of addressing the protocol. They will have to adopt what I shall call a subject-centered review strategy in which a key question to be asked is whether the research design will maximize benefit to the subject (rather than to the researcher, the researcher's institution, or even the pool of knowledge).

Some of the import of a justice-based, subject-centered review may be rather obvious. Consider a protocol that requires weekly blood samples from a group of chronically ill out-patients. The protocol might involve having patients come to the hospital weekly to give the blood. With concern for justice, which concentrates on the subjects as a least well-off group, we may be forced to ask whether it would be in the subject's interest to require that a member of the research team travel to the subject's home to obtain the sample. Of course, there might be other reasons why the chronically ill subject should come to the hospital, but justice to the least well-off may require that the patient not have to make an exhausting trip solely for the purposes of the research. This may be true even if concern for beneficence and efficient use of researcher resources supports requiring the patient to travel. In short, inconveniences to least well-off subjects become the legitimate concern in a justice-based, patient-centered review.

Thus, adding the principle of justice to the principles of beneficence and autonomy will have direct impact not only on subject selection, but research design as well. These three principles are the most central in a patient-centered ethic of research on human subjects. Other principles will from time to time be relevant as well—including the principles of truth-telling, promise-keeping, avoiding killing, and so forth. Together they will provide the framework for assessing ethical problems of research.

PART
III

Ethics in Federal Regulation

CHAPTER FIVE

Federal Regulation of Medicine and Biomedical Research: Power, Authority, and Legitimacy

With federal regulators probing every nook and cranny of what used to be the decision-making domain of the private health-care practitioner and medical researcher, it is understandable that the power, authority, and legitimacy of such regulation would be questioned. Three separate questions need to be addressed. The first is the most general: Is it legitimate in general to regulate any decisions in medicine? The second narrows the focus substantially to a rather small subset of medical decisions—those made by medical professionals: Is it legitimate to regulate decisions in medicine made by health professionals? Finally, it will be necessary to ask a question of a different order: Assuming it is legitimate to regulate some decisions made by health-care professionals, is it prudent to do so?

THE RIGHT TO REGULATE MEDICAL DECISIONS OF THE CITIZENRY

The first question may turn out to be deceptively difficult, even the hardest of the three: Does the federal government have the power, the authority, and the legitimation necessary to regulate any medical decisions at all? It is crucial to realize that the vast majority of medical decisions are not the ones that are normally thought of first as stereotypical medical decisions. The vast majority of medical decisions are made by citizens who are trained in medicine only in a rudimentary way. They are decisions made by laypeople in an effort to improve, restore, or maintain their own health or the health of significant others who are family, friends, or acquaintances. When I take aspirin for a headache, apply a band-aid to my son's cut knee, or advise a next-door neighbor to avoid breathing the exhaust from his father's car, I make medical decisions. In fact if one defines medicine as the institution in a society incorporating the beliefs, values, and practices in a society related to health and illness into social patterns and roles,[1] then countless decisions made daily by every citizen are appropriately seen as health decisions. When I decide to jog before breakfast, abstain from medicating myself with the nitrites in bacon, or help my child with his health education homework, I make medical decisions. Only the smallest fraction of medical decisions are thus made by individuals with any special medical training or skill. That has been true since the beginning of societal institutionalization of medical practices and is still true in highly technologized, professionalized cultures such as our own.

Federal regulation of medicine, then, raises the most fundamental questions of political philosophy about the power, authority, and legitimacy of the government to control the lives of individuals. The power of a well-organized, stable government to regulate personal decisions seems beyond real doubt, but also quite uninteresting from the point of view of political philosophy. I am not going to address this question of sociology or political science. The questions of authority and legitimacy are quite another matter, however.[2] If consideration of pure power is excluded—whether that be physical or psychological or economic power—we are still left with the question of whether there is a legitimate basis for governmental intervention into our daily medical decisions: our decisions to self-medicate, refuse blood transfusions, use laetrile for our cancers, use penicillin for our viral influenzas, or conduct physiological research studies on our fellow human beings without gaining the permission of some federally legitimated agency such as an institutional review board.

It is not obvious why a federal Food and Drug Administration should have the right to prohibit access to drugs simply because it has not found them to be adequately safe and effective by whatever definition of those terms and whatever set of values it has used to make such judgments.[3] Safety and efficacy are sometimes erroneously thought to be purely scientific questions to be resolved by the best pharmacological science available. No compound, however, is ever proved totally safe. At most we insist that it be safe enough given the purposes envisioned, the alternatives available, and the value of the effect anticipated. It is logically impossible to judge adequate safety without making value judgments. An experimental chemotherapeutic agent for a cancer does not have to meet the same safety requirements as a cold remedy. Safety is necessarily an evaluative judgment comparing benefits and harms envisioned.

Efficacy, likewise, is necessarily a value judgment. A compound is found effectively useful (as opposed to effectively harmful) only when the effect is a desired one. It is reported that the Spanish Pharmacopoeia describes estrogen-progesterone combinations as effective in regulating menstrual cycles, but as having a serious side effect of preventing pregnancy.

It is not easy to see why a federal agency, especially if it is staffed with professional scientists with their own sets of values and commitments, should have the authority to limit an individual citizen's right to access to such a compound simply because there is a disagreement about the value of the effects produced or the justifiability of the risks.

Federal regulation of drug use and other medical decisions by the citizen is not easy to justify. The legitimation of such regulation must be rooted in some basic societal understanding of the basic principles for the structure and function of the society. Every society will exist with some such set of principles. To the extent they are rooted in morality rather than mere power, they will reflect what has come to be called the moral point of view.[4] Rational people would agree to abide by some basic set of principles for organizing the society. Such contractual models for the establishing of a set of basic principles differ substantially over whether the task is the generation de novo of a set of principles that are an acceptable set or whether the construction is believed to reflect some underlying transcendent reality.[5] Traditionally in both religious and secular thought, the rights and responsibilities making up the basic principles have been seen as discovered— rights that humans are endowed with by their Creator or that exist in the moral laws of nature.

Regardless of the underlying metaethical assumptions, members of the society are metaphorically seen as contracting or covenanting together to abide by some basic norms or principles. In modern thought, they include principles of liberty ("compatible with like liberty for all"), equality, and the duty of promise- or contract-keeping.

It is to these basic principles that one must turn to discover if there is any legitimate basis for governmental regulation of medical decision-making. To the extent that liberty is one of those principles, the burden of proof is on those who favor federal regulation to constrain medical decisions of individuals or medical agreements among mutually consenting adults in private. If patient and physician agree among themselves that a service is to be performed at an agreed-upon fee, it is hard to see why federal government should intervene. If a private practitioner wants to purchase a CAT scanner for his office, on what grounds can a government legitimately constrain the purchase? If adult medical laypeople agree among themselves to share in providing abortion, counseling, or other "self-help" services, on what grounds can a government legitimately constrain such agreements?

But to view such societally structured medical decisions as free choices by or among isolated individuals is naive. Necessary to any plausible contractarian view of social institutions is a recognition that the society pre-exists any individual in it and shapes the very values, preferences, and opportunities available. Moreover, many, perhaps all, decisions have enormous impacts on other parties. Externalities of decisions can be great. At the very least governments are justified in constraining individual medical decisions when they have significant detrimental impacts on others. Equality of liberty requires such governmental regulation. Thus parents are given great latitude in making day-to-day medical decisions for their children, but are not given unlimited discretion. They may choose to take certain risks with their child's health. They may decide not to have an infected wound examined by a medical professional or to tolerate a child's consumption of an unhealthful diet. They may not, however, refuse a medical treatment which, if offered, would restore the child safely, simply, and surely, to reasonably normal health.[6]

Protection of the liberty and welfare of others provides the most obvious rationale for legitimate governmental intervention. It is supported by utilitarians and libertarians alike.[7] It easily justifies controls on the consumption of medicinals which, if ingested, would predictably put other parties at risk. If amphetamine consumption led predictably to violent behavior, it could justifiably be controlled. Alcohol could legitimately be controlled on account of its enormous deleterious impacts on innocent parties. Tobacco could be controlled because of its impact on passive smokers or the health-insurance money pools of public or quasi-public groups, but not, on this basis, for purely paternalistic reasons. Very few other drugs, however, have such predictable direct harmful effects on others. Their regulation on the grounds that the liberty or rights or welfare of others will be jeopardized is implausible.

Another way in which individual liberty can have a detrimental impact on others is by conveying false or misleading information. Trust is essential in the contractual relationships among individuals of a society. Federal regulations attempting to assure truthfulness in advertising and labelling are justifiable on these grounds. Regulation to assure that information is available that reasonable people would find material in deciding to use medicinals also can be seen as furthering liberty and welfare of individuals. This still does not, however, provide a basis for controlling by federal regulation access to drugs and devices for individual use, provided that they will not have predictable harmful impacts on others and provided that they have been labelled with information that is truthful and information that reasonable people would find important. Federal regulation of the use (not the labelling) of laetrile, penicillin, morphine, or anti-depressants is indeed hard, if not impossible, to justify. Control of the practicing of medicine and related services such as psychotherapy without a license is hard, if not impossible, to justify. Those who are critical of the regulation of medical professionals in clinical and research settings stand in an important libertarian tradition out of which it is very difficult to justify federal regulation for reasons other than protection of the liberty and welfare of others.

Since basic liberties may be infringed by placing constraints on individual laypeople to make medical decisions for themselves and other consenting parties, one way of preserving personal liberty while still assuring adequate information for making decisions would be to replace licensure of professionals with a certification process that provides reliable information to individuals about the qualification (or lack thereof) of any person who wants to engage in medical practices. Under the basic principle of liberty individuals would be able to make choices about how they want to be treated and by whom while still having a source of information necessary for making the choices. If one wanted to choose neurosurgery from someone trained only in hog butchering and knew what he was choosing, that decision would be permitted.

Serious problems with the replacement of licensure with certification may outweigh any of these advantages. For one, constraints would still have to be placed on practicing medicine on those who cannot consent. But if everyone had indiscriminate access to potent pharmacologicals, it would be extremely difficult to control their use on children, the mentally ill, and other non-consenting parties. Furthermore, if the privilege of practicing medicine were elevated to a right by shifting from licensure to certification, other privileges might quickly require the equivalent of licensure. The privilege of being reimbursed through governmental insurance mechanisms or obtaining the use of a governmentally funded operating room presumably should go only to those who will use the public's resources in ways acceptable to the public. Thus, while the principle of liberty might militate against licensure for purposes of self-medication and medical treatment among consenting adults at their own expense, the equivalent of licensure would be required for non-paternalistic reasons whenever the public interest or the interest of non-consenting parties was at stake.

Other basic principles of the society may also be a source of legitimation for regulation of lay medical decisions. Some principle of equity in distribution of social goods will necessarily be incorporated into a social contract that provides the basic principles of the society. In the name of providing equality of liberty, or in the name of equity more generally, some constraints on decisions by lay citizens may be justified. Some classes may have to be constrained in their medical behavior in order to prevent their choices from impacting on the medical liberties, welfare, and claims of justice of others. Society is so integrated that the isolated individual decision-maker is a mere fiction. Principles of justice may justify regulation that the principle of liberty would not.

Even purely paternalistic actions may be called for in certain situations. Prudent individuals would accept paternalistic actions on their behalf if, at some future time, they were found by some reasonable process to be incapable of acting freely, if, for instance, they became comatose or were judged by due process to be insane. They would insist on rigorous procedures so that their liberty would not be compromised when they possessed the capacity to choose in cases where only their interests were at stake. By the same token, prudent individuals would acknowledge the legitimacy of paternalistic actions on those who have been found by rigorous due process never to have been competent to act freely and competently.

Justification of federal regulation of individual medical decisions by citizens will be hard. It may not be impossible. Protection of the claims of liberty and equity of others and protection of the welfare of those who do not possess the capacity for competent decision making, may legitimate controls on medical decisions by laypeople. A society might even exercise its liberty to contract with certain groups, identified by profession or by socialization into special roles, to provide certain functions seen as essential to the common good or required by the basic principles of the society.

THE RIGHT TO REGULATE MEDICAL PROFESSIONALS

A second social contract might be established—one between the society and professional groups.[8] (For earlier suggestions of this contractual basis for the relation between the society and a profession see Veatch,[9] Pellegrino,[10] Magraw,[11] and May.[12]) While the first contract establishes the basic principles for ordering social institutions, the second would establish a relationship between the citizenry and a profession. In an exchange freely negotiated, the two groups might exchange pledges of mutual obligation in return for certain benefits that might accrue. From the liberties possessed by individuals and with the protection of the duty to keep contracts, citizens, professional and lay, may contract with one another, individually and collectively, binding one another with responsibilities and rights. These responsibilities and rights can be said to be acquired, that is acquired through individual or group action rather than derived directly from the more basic principles.[13] Society, beginning in about the late Middle Ages, began to recognize professional groups, vesting them with substantial autonomy and monopoly authority in exchange for certain responsibilities assumed by the professional group and certain benefits that would be gained by the society.[14] Provided the second social contract does not violate any of the basic principles that are the basic constitutive elements of the society itself, such private arrangements can legitimately be transacted. In the name of liberty and the right to negotiate contracts, such arrangements may be made. The rights and responsibilities of the professional group are thus derived from a second level of contract created by the society within the framework of its constitutive principles. Neophyte professionals, as they are socialized into the profession, are simultaneously socialized into the social contract establishing their rights and obligations vis-à-vis the society. The fact that each professional gains very concretely and very materially from privileges granted by the society in the funding of medical education and the protection of the exclusive right to practice the craft reinforces the basic social contract between the profession and the society as a whole. Any professional student who accepts the benefits offered by the society and the privileges of licensure explicitly affirms his acceptance of the pre-existing professional contract.

If this is the basis of professional rights and responsibility rather than some internal, more particularistic self-generated professional moral code, then the legitimation of federal regulation of medical professionals may turn out to be much easier than the legitimation of federal regulation of medical decisions made by laypeople. Laypeople are governed by the first social contract and the practices and regulations growing out of it, while medical professionals are justifiably constrained as well by their explicit commitment to practice within the framework of regulation created by the broader society in exchange for the privileges that come from being a publicly licensed professional.

Since the right to regulate licensed professionals (as opposed to laypeople or merely certified professionals) derives from this second social contract freely entered into by professionals (collectively and individually), it seems there are only two possible constraints on society's right to regulate professional medical behavior. First, the contract between the society and the profession is generated within the framework of the basic principles of the first social contract. If there are any restraints on individual and collective decision making implied by that first contract—and we have seen that it is quite hard to defend such constraints—they would place limits on the content of the contract with professionals. For instance, it is often argued that commitment to the principle of liberty makes a contract to sell oneself permanently into slavery illegitimate. If that constraint exists, a profession and the broader society would be enjoined from any contract giving the society the right to regulate professional behavior in a way that was comparable to enslavement. Permanent societal regulation of the terms, location, fees, and specialty of practice might not be an acceptable condition of the second contract if these were tantamount to having professionals sell themselves into slavery. In reality the profession is not about to agree to arrangements with the society that permit this degree of federal regulation. Lesser stipulations by society, in exchange for the rights and privileges of practicing medicine, however, are not at all incompatible with our basic commitment to liberty, equality, and contract-keeping, which presumes that free individuals will have the right to contract, as individuals and as groups, in such a way that regulation constrains their terms, location, fees, and specialty of practice. Physicians, when they agree to the terms of licensure, pledge to be bound by the regulations accompanying that license and the procedures established for changing those regulations.

A second limit on the right to regulate might be imposed by the nature of the contract between the society and the profession itself. If I am right in seeing this as a second level of social contract, then contractual agreements made between the profession and the society giving certain freedoms to the profession might themselves constrain regulation. A society could include within this contractual agreement with the profession the right to regulate fees under certain circumstances. It could also contract in such a way that it surrendered any such right during the period of the contract. Should it concede any authority to regulate in its understanding with the profession, this would remain as a limit on the right to regulate for the duration of the agreement, subject only to the prior constraints on the right to contract. If society suddenly decides it wants to regulate but has foolishly conceded its right to regulate a particular area, it finds itself in an unfortunate position of having made a bad deal.

Thus, there are only two limits on society's right to regulate licensed professionals. First, society cannot violate its own basic constitutive principles. Second, it cannot renege on previous promises made to professionals. Other than these constraints, any regulation in exchange for licensure is legitimate. Of course, if licensure were replaced by simple certification of the training and skills of citizens, society's right to regulate through the contract between the society and the profession would disappear. No contracts granting privilege and monopoly would exist, and individuals, certified or not, would be able to engage in practices limited only by the first contract.

If this is the proper understanding of the limits on the right of the government to regulate, then it will be crucial to understand the time frame of the various contracts. The rights and obligations of the original social contract appear to be without time limit. Furthermore, if society is such that all participate in the complex social institutions and the privileges of citizenship before they have the capacity to accept or reject the contract, then each individual backs into the basic principles, accepting them and acting within their framework before he ever has the chance to reflect on them. Such an individual has a limited chance to reject the principle by surrendering his citizenship, but excluding such limited opportunities for renegotiating, he is bound in perpetuity.

Other contracts arrived at within the context of the basic, enduring principles are quite another matter. Private contracts are bound by certain limits. Some kinds of commitment in perpetuity are unacceptable. It seems as if similar limits must be placed on the contract between the society and a profession. Renegotiations may be seen as taking place once in a lifetime as new professionals enter the field. This would explain the widespread use of grandfather clauses giving established professionals the right to practice in spite of the fact that they do not meet requirements of education or skill imposed on newly licensed professionals. Some pharmacists practicing today have had no more than two years of college training in spite of the fact that five years or more is now required of those being licensed today.

Another point for possible renegotiation would be at the time of license renewal. Licenses to practice are increasingly being seen as limited grants of privileges subject to renewal with imposition of reexaminations and other requirements. Possible renegotiation that would give the society the right to regulate that which it had previously surrendered might take place at the time of recertification.

Regardless of how the specific problems of renegotiation of the contract between society and the profession are solved, the notion of a second social contract entered into freely by professionals provides a very different basis of federal regulation than the basis that may exist for federal regulating of lay medical decisions. The right to regulate professional decisions in clinical and research settings seems to be very broad, indeed limited only by the constraints placed on individuals and groups to contract with one another and accept acquired rights and responsibilities.

THE WISDOM OF REGULATING MEDICAL PROFESSIONALS

The thesis that professionals are in a social contractual relationship with the larger society bound by the most basic principles of the society provides a basis for understanding the *right* of society to regulate legitimately, but it does not answer the more critical question of whether it is *prudent* for a society to regulate its professionals. Assuming at least some such regulation is prudent, it does not reveal when and how much regulation would be wise. Since our basic societal principles emphasize liberty subject to the constraints of justice, promise-keeping, and other fundamental values, it would be understandable if, whenever possible, society chose not to regulate—that is, chose not to exercise its right to regulate. It will regulate only when its basic principles require it or the general welfare necessitates it.

Consider as an example the contemporary debate about the definition of death and governmental efforts to regulate some aspects of medical professional decisions vis-à-vis the definition of death.[15] As part of the traditional arrangements between society and the profession, professionals had both the exclusive right of and the responsibility for pronouncing death. Individual professionals have been given substantial discretion for determining exactly when a person ought to be called dead and what measures ought to be used for determining that death ought to be pronounced. As long as there was virtually no debate of any practical significance, practitioners were left much to their own to make such judgments without regulation. Common law did, however, impose certain restrictions. The physician was obligated to pronounce death when, and only when, the judgment was made that all vital functions had ceased irreversibly.

The decision to call a person dead and to initiate all the social behaviors that accompany death pronouncement was essentially a social decision, not one based on medical facts. If someone had proposed to call a person dead when his brain function had irreversibly ceased even if other functions continued, there would be no biological basis for favoring one social policy over the other. No one raised that possibility; at least no one pressed it, perhaps because the distinction made no practical difference.

Once it became possible, however, to maintain other vital functions of a person whose brain had ceased functioning, the social policy choice became important. Society could have left physicians unregulated permitting them to choose to call a person dead either when the brain had ceased or when all vital functions ceased. That would have led to policy chaos, however. Society could have left to the profession the task of making the social policy choice. If so, the profession would have been acting as a surrogate for the society, not making a judgment about which its training gave it any special expertise, but acting as society's agent for the purpose of choosing among two rather plausible options for deciding when to call a person dead.

We are left with the question of when it is prudent for society to leave such judgments to the professional group trusting it to make a choice that society can accept and when it should take matters into its own hands establishing statutory law, case law, or other regulation that specifies that a person shall be called dead when certain functions cease irreversibly.

Since it is generally easier to leave matters to individuals exercising common sense than to attempt to force their behavior by regulation, it is often prudent to forego acting on the right to regulate. Two conditions make it particularly prudent for society not to regulate professional behavior. If the question at stake is believed to be one in which the profession as a whole or practitioners as individuals will reach the same decisions that the society would incorporate into regulations, then society might decide not to regulate. Unless laypeople particularly want to be involved in the actual decision making, they might cede their authority to professionals. The same decisions would result. In an earlier day, no regulation of death pronouncement was necessary because the overwhelming consensus of wise physicians differed not at all from the consensus of prudent laypeople. Individual practitioners, to be sure, might deviate just as individual people did. But it was in the profession's interest to control such deviants. Aggressive societal intervention was unnecessary.

Now, however, there is an enormous range of views on the subject.[16] Some argue the shift to a concept based on loss of brain function is too liberal,[17] while others claim that it is too conservative. They argue that it would permit some people to be considered alive who really ought to be considered dead.[18] Furthermore, since the question is one not answerable with biological or neurological evidence, disagreement also exists among medical professionals. If the distribution of the views in the medical profession followed the same pattern as that in the rest of society, then society might reasonably still leave the question to the professional group. The only thing given up by society in that case would be the right to make the decision about social policy directly.

But the pattern of distribution of views in any professional group is often not the same as in the society at large. Those choosing to enter any profession hold values that do not reflect the values of the larger society. In this case, it appears that the neurologically trained people are more willing to consider the functions of the brain to be the essentially significant functions for deciding whether a person ought to be treated as alive. Regardless of how the values held by the professional group differ from those held by the rest of society, the delegation of policy-making authority by the society to the profession on important issues when there are value differences makes no sense. It is plausible and prudent for society to regulate through its publicly legitimated authority. Society would be foolish to trust physicians' clinical intuitions on matters literally as crucial as life and death and personal freedom.

Even if there are values held by the profession that differ from those of the broader society, the society might choose to forego regulation when the issues at stake are trivial. In an earlier day, it could have required that two physicians jointly pronounce death, that an entire team of practitioners take on the task, or that certain specific procedures be used for measuring the irreversible cessation of vital functions. Although the decisions at stake were critical—literally life and death—the variation in pronouncing death that would result from imposing such regulations was not. The differences in techniques for measuring the cessation of functions would lead to differences in death pronouncement that were trivial. Society, in its wisdom, chose not to regulate such decisions. When the results will be trivial, society would often be wise not to regulate even if the professional holds values that differ from the layperson.

If, however, there is a good reason to believe that the professional group will base its decisions on a different set of values or beliefs than those held by the broader society and the differences in behavior will not be trivial, then it is foolish for society to fail to exercise its right to regulate.

This is why it makes no sense for society functioning through governmental agencies to endorse professional self-regulation and professional enforcement of their own codes of ethics. Some states regulate through licensure requiring that licenses can be suspended for unprofessional conduct. If society rather than the profession defines what is unprofessional conduct, that is reasonable, but the term implies that the limits of acceptable behavior will be defined by the profession and its code. Some states mistakenly turn over to the professional organization or to members of the profession, adjudication of questions of professional misconduct. It is essential to a profession that it generate its own code based on values and commitments internal to the profession.[19] A professional code is, thus, radically different from a contract or covenant negotiated between the society and the profession.[20] A code is an autonomously generated summary of the standards embraced by a group based on its own, often particularistic values. No justification to the broader society is necessary. It is not even possible according to many views of professional ethics.

To the extent that a professional code is based on professionally held values rather than publicly held ones and to the extent the value differences are significant and the resulting behavioral differences are not trivial, society is foolish if it legitimates enforcement of the profession's code rather than the social contracts providing the basic principles for organizing the society's institutions and the relationship of laypeople with professionals.

Under these circumstances it is a mistake for society to cede to the professional group the authority to determine the concept of death used for pronouncing a person dead. It is especially foolish if there is any evidence that the professional group as a whole holds philosophical, religious, or other evaluative positions that differ from the broader society.

There is substantial evidence that on many crucial philosophical and ethical questions the profession does differ from the broader society. Since decisions, if left to professionals, would impact directly on non-professionals, we have precisely the circumstances where society ought to regulate the profession in mandating the concept of death to be used by professionals. No professional need be bound by such societal regulation. He has the option, under normal circumstances, of ceasing to be bound by the contract by the society and the profession. But then he must surrender his privileges as well as his obligations.

A similar analysis explains why society has the authority to impose regulations on professionals in the prescribing of drugs. Society does not permit a physician to prescribe heroin—no matter what we may think of society's judgment and no matter what individual practitioners may think about the humaneness of using heroin in caring for terminal cancer patients. If society holds values that it considers central and if it believes individual practitioners or the profession as a whole holds different values, it has the right to regulate medical practitioners. It also would be wise in doing so.

If society would be wise in regulating the behavior of professionals, it would be foolish to delegate to those professionals or some of their group the authority to make the key evaluative choices. The FDA, for example, should be seen as an arm of social policy. To the extent that it imposes restriction on the behavior of laypeople who are citizens, it must confront the arguments against the right of the society to regulate the medical decisions of individual citizens. Its legitimacy in regulating health professionals' decisions to use unapproved drugs or use approved drugs for unapproved uses is a totally different matter. It has the right to control practitioners' behavior and is wise in doing so whenever there is reason to fear that practitioners will act on values that differ significantly from those of the larger society and when the behavioral results will be other than trivial.

At the same time, if the FDA is an agency of society that may legitimately regulate professionals and possibly may even legitimately regulate the behavior of lay citizens, it is a mistake to turn over the decision making of such an agency to professionals used to staff it. The FDA is, and ought to be, a political animal regulating professionals and laypeople in ways based on societally held values within the constraints of the basic principles of the social contract. Society as a whole may hold different values about risk-taking in the use of saccharin or level of certainty in evaluating evidence about the use of laetrile. They may hold different values regarding the benefits and harms of the alternatives to these chemicals.

Federal regulations requiring consent for the use of human subjects for medical research can be defended on the same basis. All ought to recognize that there are disutilities of requiring consent. They exist especially in those rare cases when researchers believe they have good reason for not getting consent. It seems, however, that the fact that a researcher believes consent should not be obtained is not enough reason for society to forego a regulation requiring consent. The difference in perception regarding a requirement of consent may be accounted for on a number of bases.

Some may argue that medical professionals cannot be trusted to act with good will in the absence of regulation. There is some evidence that some researchers are lacking in good will.[21] That, by itself, however, does not seem to be an adequate reason for justifying regulation. In the first place, the number of researchers lacking good will is small. Almost never have I encountered outright evil intent on the part of either researchers or clinicians. Even if practitioners lacking good will did exist, the interests in the profession in controlling those that were so outrageously malevolent might be great enough to motivate intra-professional regulation. That mechanism has worked successfully in dealing with a small number of seriously malevolent practitioners. If lack of good will were the problem, elaborate regulations requiring consent or other standards of professional conduct might be expendable.

That is not the problem, however. The real problem is difference in basic value commitment. Clinicians are traditionally committed to doing what they think will benefit their patients. Researchers are uniquely committed to doing what they think will produce the greatest good. With some exceptions both groups have a good record of acting in good faith on those commitments. But neither value commitment corresponds with the values of the broader society committed to liberty, equality, fidelity to promises, and a set of values quite alien to traditional professional ethics.

The alternative to federal regulation on questions such as consent is reliance on the well-intentioned intuition of a group whose individual judgments may, to some extent, be based on values that differ significantly from those who value self-determination. If the lay population relied on professional judgment of those not seeing self-determination as inherently critical, the citizens' right to self-determination would be violated, at least in certain cases. It would be violated in all clinical cases where physicians were committed to serving the patient's interest and believed it was in the patient's interest not to get consent. It would also be violated in all research cases where researchers were committed uniquely to the principle of producing the greater good on balance and thought that on balance greater good would be served by not getting consent. The only prudent course when professionals are given authority to act and yet are believed to hold values differing from those upon which they must act is for society to enact regulations requiring the behaviors valued by laypeople, such as getting consent.

The final stand for those who oppose federal regulation might well be a retreat to the fact/value distinction which claims that at least in technical areas of medicine, regulators ought to refrain from regulating. Sophisticated professionals might concede that many FDA decisions are really judgments based on values or on commitments to ethical principles such as liberty. They might concede that obtaining consent in problematic cases will depend on whether one values self-determination or wants to maximize benefits to the patient or society. They might concede that the basic conceptual questions about when to call a person dead are essentially philosophical, that no medical training helps one decide whether to call a person dead when his neurological function or circulatory function ceases irreversibly. They might accept the legitimacy of regulation in these areas.

They might still hold out, however, for freedom from regulation in more technical areas such as deciding whether there is any evidence of tumor regression after laetrile testing, whether there will be psychological harm from informing a patient he is in a cancer chemotherapy protocol, or whether in using a electroencephalogram for measuring the irreversible loss of brain function the period of testing ought to be 24 hours or whether it can be reduced to six hours or one hour or even dispensed with entirely. These, at least, they argue, are purely scientific questions that should remain outside the grasp of the federal regulators and safely tucked into the protecting arms of the professional group with scientific expertise in the area.

The prudent society will normally leave such technical questions free from regulation. But even these questions are not totally outside the rational oversight of the broader society in situations where significant social policy decisions must be made based on such seemingly purely scientific or technical questions. It is increasingly recognized that no scientific questions totally escape evaluative, ethical, metaethical, and metaphysical assumptions. Occasionally, basic questions of value or world view, basic philosophical assumptions, or underlying systems of theory and belief will significantly impinge on judgments that at first seem purely technical. It is impossible to prove that laetrile does not cure cancer, only that evidence at an acceptable level of confidence seems to reasonable people to lead to the conclusion it is useless. Judgments based on philosophical and other beliefs and values will necessarily enter these evaluations at the point of deciding what level of confidence is acceptable, what constitutes reasonableness, and what outcomes are useless. The broader society should be aware that if it defers judgments even in these technical matters to professional experts, there is a risk that a judgment will be made that would not have been made by laypeople if, by some miraculous transposition, they were to gain the knowledge of the experts and retain the values they now hold as laypeople. Fortunately, this need not often be a problem. The risks of public intervention in such areas through federal regulation may produce more harm than good. The same criteria emerge, however, as in instances when a decision must be made by society whether to regulate professionals in their policy-making roles. If basic values differ significantly and the questions being asked are not trivial, then the public should be concerned about the possibility that even on apparently technical matters judgments may be made that would not have been made by laypeople holding differing values. In such cases federal regulation may turn out to be a prudent protection. The risks of such intervention, especially in the areas normally thought of as the scientific domain, are great. It is not illogical, however, for the public to insist on such regulation as part of its social contract with the profession.

CHAPTER SIX

Federal Regulations: Progress and Problems

On January 26, 1981, the Department of Health and Human Services (DHHS) published its long-awaited final regulations amending current agency policy governing research involving human subjects.[1] DHHS regulations, at least until now, have come to be taken as the legal, and often the moral, standard for protecting human subjects in the United States. These regulations require that, with certain exemptions, all research involving human subjects conducted by DHHS or funded in whole or in part by DHHS be reviewed by an IRB. The regulations lay down the requirements for IRB membership and criteria for approval of research. Rules regulating IRB membership require that the board have at least five members and that they not be entirely one profession or sex. At least one member must have no affiliation with the institution. In order for research to be approved, the approval of the majority of voters present at that meeting must be attained. Seven criteria for approval must be met.

1. Sound Research Design. One requirement is that procedures be consistent with sound research design. The point is an obvious one. If a procedure exposing a subject to risk is one that cannot produce any useful knowledge, the risk is morally unjustified. Of course, though necessary, this criterion is not sufficient to justify research. It is not acceptable, for instance, to argue for a research design that violates the rights of subjects rather than for one that does not simply because the design violating the subject's rights is more elegant or will produce better data. Other moral criteria must be met as well.

2. Protection of Privacy and Confidentiality. The protection of subject's privacy and confidentiality is critical for any research. In most projects, protection of confidentiality is routine, posing no significant problems for research design.

3. *Equity in Treatment of Subjects*. The DHHS regulations require that subject selection be equitable. This means that any research that targeted its subjects for the poor, for clinic patients, or for those of minority or other vulnerable groups, would have a difficult time meeting the criterion of equity. As a rule it is also bad science to bias one's subject sample by selecting for special groups of this sort.

4. *Benefit/Harm Considerations*. The remaining criteria for approval have the potential of raising important problems for research design. The first of these relates directly to the broad ethical principle of beneficence: "Risks to subjects are reasonable in relation to anticipated benefits, if any, to subjects, and the importance of the knowledge that may reasonably be expected to result."[2] A second is closer to the notions of autonomy and equity in that it focuses exclusively on the ethical claims of the individual subject: Benefits are limited exclusively to the subjects of the research. For example, this implies that in a randomized clinical trial for both the experimental and control arms of a study, the predicted ratio of subject benefit to subject harm must be similar for the arms.

5. *Data Monitoring*. A fifth criterion for IRB approval is the requirement that the "research plan must make adequate provisions for monitoring the data collected to ensure safety of subjects."[3] This is required so that research can be stopped if unanticipated harms occur or if the needed level of statistical significance has been reached.

6. *Informed Consent Will Be Appropriately Documented*. This is a straightforward requirement specifying regulations on various ways informed consent may be documented.

7. *Informed Consent Will Be Sought from Each Prospective Subject or the Subject's Legally Authorized Representative*. Eight basic elements of consent are specified which, save for certain exceptions, must be met:[4]

(1) A statement that the study involves research, an explanation of the purposes of the research and the expected duration of the subject's participation, a description of the procedures followed, and identification of any procedures which are experimental;

(2) A description of any reasonably foreseeable risks or discomforts to the subject;

(3) A description of any benefits to the subject or to others which may reasonably be expected from the research;

(4) A disclosure of appropriate alternative procedures or courses of treatment, if any, that might be advantageous to the subject;

(5) A statement describing the extent, if any, to which confidentiality of records identifying the subject will be maintained;

(6) For research involving more than minimal risk, an explanation as to whether any compensation and an explanation as to whether any medical treatments are available if injury occurs and, if so, what they consist of, or where further information may be obtained;

(7) An explanation of whom to contact for answers to pertinent questions about the research and research subjects' rights, and whom to

contact in the event of a research-related injury to the subject; and

(8)   A statement that participation is voluntary, refusal to participate will involve no penalty or loss of benefits to which the subject is otherwise entitled, and the subject may discontinue participation at any time without penalty or loss of benefits to which the subject is otherwise entitled.

We shall examine the adequacy of these regulations in this chapter. A helpful way to begin to see any flaws they have is to consider that all the following hypothetical research projects would presumably be permitted according to the 1981 regulations:

—My neighbor, who is an employee of a local mental health center, will be able to read my psychiatric record for research purposes without my permission, provided he does not record any information in a manner that identifies me.

—I may, in interviews, ask high school students potentially stressful or embarrassing questions about their sexual behavior, recording responses so that the subjects can be identified, provided I do not deal with topics where students' responses could reasonably place them at risk of criminal or civil liability.

—A researcher may take a woman's uterus removed during surgery and display it in his laboratory for research purposes without the woman knowing about it, provided her name is not identified with the tissue.

—If I want to study the reasons young, pregnant, unmarried women choose to have their babies rather than abort them so that I can develop psychological strategies for convincing other young women to abort, provided I do not identify them in my data, I may search their records without their permission. I may do so even though I have reason to believe that the women whose records I am using oppose abortion and would seriously object to the purposes of my research.

—A military scientist wanting to understand human response to military authority may deceive subjects by making them think they are inflicting death-producing punishment even though doing so could cause psychological damage to the subjects. He may do so provided the research is judged (presumably by the researcher) to involve no more than minimal risk, and provided certain other conditions are met, including appropriate debriefing after the research.

Before examining the flaws in the regulations that these hypothetical examples reveal, it is first necessary to have an understanding of the history of the regulations.

HISTORICAL DEVELOPMENT

The first formal review procedures were developed in 1953 in connection with the opening of the National Institutes of Health's (NIH's) Clinical Center. More critical, however, was the 1966 Public Health Service requirement that clinical research could be supported only if "the judgment of the investigator is subject to prior review by his institutional associates. . . ." Although federal (departmental) guidelines had existed since the late 1960s,[5] the contemporary regulatory effort to revise and tighten the protection of citizens who are exposed to research risks began in 1973 soon after public disclosure of studies such as the Tuskegee Study. In this study, patients who were primarily poor and black were purposely not given treatment for syphilis so that the "natural" course of the disease could be studied.

The public outcry led to hearings of the Subcommittee on Health of the Senate Committee on Labor and Public Welfare. I had the privilege of working with subcommittee staff in planning those hearings and then testifying before the subcommittee. Following the model of Henry Beecher's 1966 *New England Journal* critique of research ethics, I developed a collection of 43 research protocols published since 1966 that were ethically suspect. These were presented to the subcommittee. In all 43 cases the research was done in the United States or the funding came from this country. They included—to mention only a few—administering LSD to subjects without informing them of the risks (subjects were paid $2.00 per hour to participate), requiring institutionalized mental patients to tend crops under the possible threat of attack of the Viet Cong (patients not "volunteering" for this study were given unmodified electric shock "therapy" and then, if unsuccessful, were denied food up to three days) in a behavior modification experiment, intentionally exposing children suffering from asthma to "challenge doses" of antigens known to produce attacks, and exposing subjects to pain experiments during what they thought were regular medical check-ups in a study on age, sex, and racial differences in pain tolerance.[6] Others testifying also provided evidence that more careful protection of human subjects was needed.[7] These hearings gave rise to The National Research Act, passed in 1974, which established the National Commission for the Protection of Human Subjects of Biomedical and Behavioral Research. The human experimentation committees, which had existed previously at many institutions, were, in the 1974 Act, designated institutional review boards (IRBs). The National Commission reviewed the adequacy of this protection and published in between 1975 and 1978 four special reports on particular groups: human fetuses,[8] prisoners,[9] children,[10] and those institutionalized as mentally infirm,[11] as well as a report on IRBs[12] and a report on basic ethical principles (The Belmont Report).[13] All of these reports recommend continued use of the existing mechanism of an IRB to review research. In ethically difficult cases the reports recommended that the IRB be supplemented by an additional review by a national ethical advisory body, a group that existed for a brief time (1978–1980). The Commission's recommendations on the IRB were published November 30, 1978. The Secretary of Health and Human Services was required by law to respond within 180 days, indicating whether the recommendations were appropriate, and, if not, to publish an adequate statement of the reasons for his determination. A proposed set of regulations did not appear until August 14, 1979; and final action was not taken until January, 1981, over two years after the original request for a response.

In many respects the Commission's work was monumental. Never before had a governmental body been devoted primarily to examining the ethical issues of a public policy. The Commission produced a thorough examination of the issues—as well as an important model for further efforts in ethics and public policy. Many of the Commission's recommendations were accepted by the DHHS. Yet despite these accomplishments, as seen from the hypothetical research protocols presented earlier, there is still room for some further improvement.

PROBLEMS REMAINING WITH THE REGULATIONS

The Scope of the Regulations

Before the National Commission wrote its recommendations (published between 1975 and 1978), the Department of Health, Education, and Welfare (DHEW) regulations were ambiguous in stating which federal entities were within DHEW's regulatory authority. The writers of the 1973 DHEW regulations stated that the regulations applied to grants and contracts funded by DHEW, but the National Research Act, which mandated such review in the first place, had stated that no grants and contracts could be awarded unless the institution had an IRB reviewing *all* human research conducted at or sponsored by it. This led to a confusing situation. Although DHEW policy dominated, there were no fewer than twenty-eight federal entities that conducted or supported human research outside DHEW's regulatory authority. These included not only controversial research by the Army, Navy, Air Force, and the intelligence community, but the Bureau of Standards, the Department of Agriculture, and the Federal Railroad Administration. Of these, nine had no formal policies protecting human subjects. Of the others, four adopted the DHEW regulations with no modifications, but others adopted them with various changes. The result was different and sometimes incompatible regulations. Thus, the Commission's first recommendation was to cut through this confusion by proposing that regulations under DHEW jurisdiction apply to all research involving human subjects covered by federal regulation. Had this requirement been accepted, it might still have excluded some research conducted by individuals totally escaping federal funding or regulation. Some of the most controversial research had in fact been done in such settings; but virtually all mainstream research, had this recommendation been accepted, would have fallen under a much simplified and more consistent set of regulations. Research covered by federal regulation (such as privately funded, FDA-regulated drug research) and research supported by other federal agencies besides DHEW would have been included.

Unfortunately, the Commission's recommendation was not accepted by the DHHS. Because of a last-minute change in the 1981 regulations that excluded all research not conducted or funded by the DHHS, even the kinds of unethical research the regulations were originally designed to prevent could be conducted without DHHS regulatory scrutiny or sanction. One need only recall the Willowbrook or Tuskegee studies or the studies presented to Congress in 1973 to see the possible results. If researchers are only shrewd enough to conduct this type of study without using DHHS funds, their experiments could escape the body of regulations that has much improved the moral and scientific climate of research involving human subjects. It is only on a voluntary basis or on the basis of state law that institutions subject their non-federally funded research to the regulatory standards. Fortunately, reputable institutions have normally imposed this requirement and other federal agencies—such as the FDA—have made an effort to bring their regulations in line. Though, of course, most researchers have good intentions and though many hold roughly the same values as those of the rest of society, there will always be a minority of researchers who do not have what most people would consider to be good intentions or moral integrity, and there will always be researchers, though admittedly with good intentions, who do not share the same values society has in general. Protection is needed whether it be through government regulation or from some other source.

An argument can be made that government protection is preferable since society would agree to give up some freedoms (such as a researcher's liberty to conduct studies as he or she sees fit) in return for the overall protection of its citizens. This argument would be consistent with the now well-known view that a just society can be arrived at by imagining what citizens would agree to in making a contract with the government, because one actually knew his or her role or status in society.[14] I would support this type of Rawlsian justification for requiring government control over research ethics. The Commission's recommendation was a wise one.

Yet since the watchword of late is government deregulation, we shall have to look beyond the federal regulatory process. At best this will mean a new sense of responsiblity for other groups, individuals, and government bodies, because all research not funded by DHHS is outside the scope of its regulation. The research institutions of the country will have to take up some of the slack. Normally they are charged with the administration of the IRB, and they continue to have the authority to make HHS standards or even more rigorous standards mandatory for all research in their institutions. They should, I believe, immediately require that all research involving human subjects exempted from HHS regulations be made subject to the IRB's new expedited review process or to full IRB scrutiny. The IRB will then be able to assess quickly whether problems of confidentiality or objection to purpose could plausibly arise and to provide an independent judgment of risks. Institutions should feel compelled to protect their own integrity.

Other public agencies will also have a new responsibility. In some states, such as New York, laws are already in force making all research not subject to HHS regulation subject to state authority, which implies very similar standards.[15] State, county, and city governments may have to fill the void to protect subjects adequately, by extending HHS-type regulations to institutions within their jurisdiction.

REVIEWING NO-RISK AND MINIMUM-RISK RESEARCH

Another DHEW requirement that was in effect before the Commission's recommendations were put forth was that IRBs were required to assure that the research meet the criteria that subjects' rights are protected and adequate consent is obtained. For some reason, however, this review was required only if the IRB first had determined that subjects were at risk. Protocols that did not place subjects at risk could thus escape review even if the subject matter was sensitive and subjects might have good reason for refusing to consent. Obviously if such a subject were not placed at risk, the IRB would not, according to the regulations, examine questions of subject rights or consent. Adopting the Commission's first recommendation, that DHEW regulations apply to all research involving human subjects covered by federal regulations, could have solved this problem. However, instead of eliminating problems posed by the DHEW regulations, the Commission may have backed into the same difficulties by its definition of human subjects and by specifying conditions when consent need not be obtained. The Commission defined "human subject" as "a person about whom an investigator . . . conducting scientific research obtains (1) data through intervention or interaction with the person, or (2) identifiable private information."[16] Thus, evidently consent would not be required if the subject was not identifiable—e.g., data from the subject's medical record with the name concealed—even if the research is likely to be objectionable to a great number of persons.

The 1981 DHHS regulations, the ones now in effect, adopt the same definition, in addition limiting the term "human subject" to living individuals.[17] This has the potential of permitting researchers to gain access to sensitive medical records of deceased persons without the benefit of regulatory protection or IRB review. In addition, the 1981 regulations further limit regulatory protection and IRB review by following the Commission's recommendation of creating whole categories of research that are exempt. Generally, they are categories that pose minimum risk provided certain requirements are met. The regulation writers have heard the powerful voices of those who want to pursue studies that are commonly believed to have remote, minimal, or nonexistent risks. Examples of these types of studies are education experiments, surveys, interviews, and studies involving observation of public behavior.

However, although these categories of studies appear to be innocuous, some of them can pose ethical problems warranting IRB attention. Some of these studies are potentially harmful. The interviews with high school students about their sexual behaviors is an example of possibly risky research that is exempt from even expedited review. Even if these studies pose no risk of harm (physical or psychological), the subjects' rights may still be violated. Respect for persons might still require that subjects have a right to consent, even if they are not at risk. The woman whose therapeutically removed uterus would be on display in the lab, for example, might want a chance to say "yes" to the researcher, even if she is not in any danger. The person whose mental health records are searched by his neighbor might still want his privacy protected, even if he will not be identified with the information any further and even if he is not at risk.

For consent to be adequately informed, the subject must have been given an explanation of the purposes of the research. Possibly the young women who had refused abortion would want to know the purpose of the research and even if they themselves were at no risk to have a chance to say "no" to the study designed to find strategies to encourage other young women to abort. Furthermore, respect for persons seems to cease with death since the regulations apply only to living subjects, apparently excluding research on cadavers or autopsy parts. The Uniform Anatomical Gift Act may require continued respect for what once was a person, but the DHHS regulations do not.

Though the principle of autonomy requiring respect for persons' freedom that grounds the informed-consent requirement is generally carefully protected by the DHHS, this is one area in which the DHHS mistakenly allows consequentialistic considerations (i.e., the goal of research gains) to override respect for autonomy, privacy, and other moral concerns beyond the benefits of the research. The result of the 1981 regulations is that, by creating exempted categories of research, the DHHS exposes subjects to the serious possibility that their rights will be violated just as they were under the older 1973 regulations that straightforwardly excluded risk-free research.

EXPEDITED REVIEWS

A third change in regulations recommended by the Commission is that expedited reviews be provided for studies involving no more than minimal risk and no violation of the basic ethical principles governing research involving human subjects. No formal authorization had existed previous to the Commission's recommendations to speed up review of routine, non-controversial protocols even though about two-thirds of the existing IRBs at the time had some procedure for screening out noncontroversial protocols. The 1981 DHHS regulations did incorporate this recommendation thus allowing for uniform minimal standards for expediting these reviews. Some examples of research that is currently approved for expedited review are studies on hair, nail clippings, teeth, excreta, saliva, placentas, and other easily obtained body wastes as well as noninvasive procedures such as weight recordings.[18] No IRB is required to expedite reviews in these approved categories though most do. Some of the more sophisticated IRBs will identify certain research within their institutions where, because of the nature of the research or the investigator's past record, full review is routinely required even though the proposed research falls in an expedited category. When expedited review is conducted, either individuals or subcommittees are assigned to do the review. This to some extent alleviates the problems such as possible consent violations discussed in the last paragraph. While risk-free and minimal-risk research posing these problems might slip through existing review procedures due to exemptions, if expedited review were required for all research including that currently exempt and if it were working correctly, the problems could be flagged by the reviewer and sent to the full committee.

CONSIDERING LONG-TERM EFFECTS

A fourth area of concern is seen in the Commission recommendation that "the possible long-range effects of applying knowledge gained in the research (e.g., the possible effects of the research on public policy . . .) should not be considered as among those research risks falling within the purview of the IRB. . . ."[19] It is interesting that the DHHS accepted this recommendation since it seems to be very unclear what is intended to be excluded.

Perhaps what is meant are very remote consequences such as changes in public opinion toward research or possible public-policy controversies. But what would follow logically, as worded, is that long-term benefits to society (as opposed to the subject) of, for example, a chemotherapy protocol (e.g., cancer being cured or survival rates increased) cannot be taken into account. If that is so, it is unclear how one could ever justify research. Research is usually justified by the importance of the knowledge to be gained. And presumably some of that importance will be expressed in terms of the long-term effects on society of possible successes. Thus, in light of their known intentions, it is a mystery both why the Commission came up with this recommendation in the first place and why it was incorporated by the DHHS into its regulations.

Another logical consequence of the DHHS statement is that long-term risks are not to be considered. It may be that this is what the Commission and DHHS meant to exclude in their statement. Perhaps they were attempting to guard against over-conservative thinking. Nevertheless, as it is worded, this regulation is unreasonable since it would be imprudent never to consider long-term risks. For example, long-term risks in drug studies such as genetic risks to future generations are imperative considerations.

ADDING EQUITY AS A PRINCIPLE

A fifth area of concern is seen in the Commission recommendation that the principle of equity be applied in determining what constitutes ethical research. This was discussed in its Belmont Report as well as the IRB Report. This was the first time that such concerns found their way into governmental documents on human-subjects research. The recommendations stated bluntly that the selection of subjects must be equitable. Although there had been much concern over children and mentally ill patients, relatively little attention had been given to the poor as a vulnerable group of potential research subjects. The Commission recommended that researchers have to justify any proposed involvement of hospitalized patients, other institutionalized persons, or disproportionate numbers of racial or ethnic minorities or persons of low socioeconomic status. The Commission was very short on specifics—it did not provide criteria for what would count as an adequate justification, but this initial effort to move beyond traditional ethics of benefit, harm, and consent in research was promising indeed. The current DHHS regulations are much improved because of their acceptance of this important innovation in the ethical underpinnings of the new regulations.

Yet they still limit the concern about equity to the *selection* of subjects when that concern might extend much further. IRBs might insist, for example, that justice or equity be taken into account in designing the research itself. Benefits must be apportioned between subjects and others as research is designed. If subjects are particularly poorly off, for example, equity might require more willingness to sacrifice some societal benefits to make sure subject welfare is maximized. We shall see how equity becomes a serious consideration in research design in chapter 9.

Also, the question of equity forces us to deal with the moral responsibility of the researchers to the losers in a randomization. What responsibility, if any, do researchers retain for assuring that those who are randomized into a less effective treatment regimen are given high priority for receiving the treatment that through the course of the study proves to be more effective? Equity requires that special consideration be given to subjects both in their selection and in the design of the research so as to maximize the subject's welfare. Although this can create serious problems for research design, the problems should not be insurmountable.

CONSENT REQUIREMENTS

Next, the Commission recommended significant revisions of the consent requirements. The most important was the explicit formulation of the standard for deciding how much information must be transmitted for consent to be informed. Confusion had existed over whether the standard ought to be that subjects be told enough information to protect their interests or whether they should have information to exercise autonomous decision making. The problem arises most dramatically when a researcher believes some significant information is potentially harmful or disturbing to the subject. The Commission recommendations followed the line of judicial decisions over the past decade (outlined in chapter 3) that emphasize the priority of self-determination. They called for communicating information that subjects may reasonably be expected to desire in considering whether to participate in the research. The courts have made it clear that the standard is what reasonable persons in the subject's circumstance would want to know (i.e., would find material) rather than what reasonable professionals who happen to be IRB

members would desire. The Commission's recommendations made clear that
the standard no longer could be what IRB members would want to know. But
in adopting the standard of what subjects would reasonably be expected to
desire, it still does not sufficiently clarify who ought to do the expecting.
More explicit emphasis on the potential difference between the judgments of
IRB members and subjects about what subjects may reasonably be expected
to desire would have been helpful. As part of the consent debate, the
Commission considerably advanced the discussion of steps that can be taken
to assure that consent is really informed and voluntary. They suggested such
practical steps as providing an interval of time in which to weigh risks and
consider alternatives before the research begins, avoiding asking for consent
when subjects are in a vulnerable emotional state, limiting remuneration,
and taking special care in using students as subjects.

One improvement suggested was the explicit specification that subjects
be told who is conducting the study, who is funding it, who should be
contacted if harm occurs, and whether treatment or compensation is available if harm occurs. (Here there was agreement between the Commission
and the Department of HEW, which had just issued interim regulations
requiring that the policy regarding compensation be conveyed to subjects.)
It is remarkable that previous regulations failed to make explicit that possible
compensation mechanisms or the absence thereof would reasonably be material to subjects in deciding whether to consent.

Most of these recommendations have been incorporated into the current
DHHS regulations. They state, for example:

> An investigator shall seek . . . consent only under circumstances that
> provide the prospective subject . . . sufficient opportunity to consider
> whether or not to participate and that minimize the possibility of coercion
> or undue influence. The information that is given . . . shall be in language
> understandable to the subject. . . .[20]

Further, the list of elements for an adequately informed consent has
been significantly expanded. Subjects must now be given the name of a
person to contact for answers to questions or in the event of a research-
related injury. They must be told of additional costs that may result from
research participation. They must be told of significant new findings developed during the course of the research that may relate to their willingness
to continue to participate. When faithfully put into practice, this requirement makes it difficult to get subjects to complete studies if it appears that
they are in a group getting comparatively poor results, but a reasonable
subject is likely to find this information crucial to his or her decision to
continue to participate. (This is the problem of preliminary data taken up in
chapter 11.) The current regulations even call for one general requirement
for informed consent that the Commission did not suggest, namely that no
waivers of the subject's legal rights to release the investigator, the sponsor,

the institution, or its agents from liability for negligence could be permitted.[21] Though the above changes are significant improvements in the consent requirement, some problems remain in the current regulations concerning when the requirement to obtain informed consent may be waived or altered.

The Problem of Deception

Before the Commission's recommendations were published, DHEW regulations placed limits on waivers of consent that were extreme and would not normally allow either consideration of benefit to the patient or benefit to the research to justify waiving consent. In contrast, the Commission recommendations vacillated. They said, "The IRB can approve withholding or altering of . . . information provided it determines that the incomplete disclosure or deception is not likely to be harmful in and of itself and that sufficient information will be disclosed to give subjects a fair opportunity to decide whether they want to participate in that research."[22] This was hard to interpret in light of the prior commitment that consent must be based on information that subjects may reasonably be expected to desire in considering whether to participate. Since the purpose of the experiment is one of the elements identified, apparently the only tolerable deceptions about purpose that the IRB can justify would be ones that subjects would not reasonably want to know in the first place. This might call for such techniques as having researchers draw samples of surrogate subjects, explaining the research plan, and asking them whether they would have desired to know the purpose of the research before consenting. Since some people will object in principle to deception in this way, such evidence would be hard to come by. In that case the door that would seem to be opened to deception in research would only be a mirage. The only acceptable deceptions, in spite of the Commission's apparent opening, would seem to be cases where subjects somehow consent to being deceived or would not object to being deceived. Such consents that do not invalidate the research are conceivable but unlikely.

Unfortunately, the 1981 regulations, because of their acceptance of virtually all the Commission's recommendations on this topic, share these difficulties. The 1981 regulations state that consent may be waived or the requirements altered if the study involves no more than minimal risk, the waiver or alteration will not adversely affect the rights and welfare of the subjects, if the research could not practicably be carried out without the waiver, and if appropriate, subjects are provided with additional pertinent information after participation.[23] The 1981 regulations also seem to accept the Commission's recommendation that consent be based on information that subjects may reasonably be expected to desire: "An investigator shall seek . . . consent only under circumstances that provide the prospective subject . . . sufficient opportunity to consider whether or not to participate. . . ."[24] The DHHS, as we have seen, also includes a statement of the purpose of the study as one of the elements of consent. Thus we have the same problem:

The only tolerable deceptions are ones in which subjects would not object to being deceived.

Further, the current regulations on the consent requirement contain a puzzling and potentially dangerous provision, which we have already seen, that may subordinate the principle of respect for persons to the consequentialistic aim of the pursuit of research benefit. This is the provision that exempts research from the requirement of informed consent when it could not practicably be carried out without the waiver. Deception research would, according to this provision, seem to be justified. The argument for the waiver is essentially: "Respecting subjects' rights to consent will destroy the experiment." In other words, when benefits clash inevitably with respect for persons' rights, the benefits take precedent. This is consequentialist reasoning of the crudest kind. To be fair, the other conditions listed for acceptable waivers or alterations of the consent requirement must be met. Yet as we will see it may be that these provisions are not consistent with one another.

The final—and also puzzling—provision for acceptable consent waivers or alterations is the one added by the Secretary of HHS to the National Commission's proposal. This is the provision in the 1981 regulations that states that waiving consent is acceptable provided that it will not adversely affect the rights and welfare of the subjects. Yet it is virtually impossible to do deception research without potential violation of rights. Consenting to participate in someone else's research project for someone else's purposes is precisely what is required by respect for persons. No deception researcher can be sure that he or she is proposing a waiver of consent in a manner that does not violate the rights of a number of potential subjects. How could researchers possibly know whether subjects would object to a particular study unless they ask them (i.e., obtain consent)? Perhaps it could be answered that the researcher should decide based upon how the average person would feel about the deception. Yet the principle of autonomy does not require respect for persons "as a group" but quite clearly requires respect for each individual's freedom of choice. The principle of autonomy cannot be applied in terms of a general class of persons. It is coherent only if applied at the level of each individual person. If this reasoning is accepted, no waivers under this provision would ever be possible without explicit justification. I hope that is the way the provision is interpreted, but I suspect it will not be. Any other alternative subordinates respect for persons totally to considerations of the benefits of the research. The only way around the problem of withholding information when such withholding is essential to the nature of the study is to attempt to use some mechanism whereby consent can actually be obtained or can be contracted. In some populations providing ongoing groups who are potential research subjects—groups such as students or employees or institution residents—a blanket consent could be obtained from some persons who would be willing to be deceived in some future studies. Possibly this could be done without biasing the results of future deception research. If it were, then the problem would be solved. In other cases it might be possible, using surrogate panels such as those described in chapter 12, to argue that reasonable subjects would not want to know about the purpose of the research and the presence of the deception.

Excluding Consent by Defining Subjects Too Narrowly

Another problem in the 1981 regulations concerning waivers of obtaining consent lies in the DHHS's definition—accepted from the Commission's recommendation—of "human subject." As we have seen, the DHHS defines "human subjects" in such a way that individuals on whom research is done who cannot be identified are not included in the definition.[25] It seems strange indeed that persons upon whom there are medical files containing identifiers are subjects and the mere deletion of identifiers can make them non-subjects. If the individuals provide data essential to the study, it seems they are the subjects of the study whether identified or not. Examining medical records is an invasion of privacy that is the moral equivalent of wiretapping. It would be more reasonable to admit that such persons are still subjects, but that no IRB review is needed and no consent required (if that is the policy the DHHS favors).

Waiving consent in these cases is, it seems to me, much more problematic than is realized. The presumption appears to be that the only reason persons would want to have a consent procedure is to protect themselves against harm or to protect confidentiality. Why, then, must subjects, when they are asked to consent, be told the purposes of the study? If subjects are to be viewed as autonomous individuals capable of making choices about whether they want to participate in a particular study, the mere fact that they will not be harmed and will not be identified should not disqualify them from having the opportunity to consent.

Persons could unwittingly become part of several studies under these recommendations and definitions, ones to which they quite plausibly could have serious objections. A record search attempting to correlate race, IQ, and some obscure blood factor would not require consent. If the individuals were not identified in the records, they would not even be subjects. Consider the hypothetical study referred to earlier. A gynecological clinic could have psychological profiles on unwed pregnant women. A researcher may want to study the psychological characteristics of those who chose bear their children rather than abort. The researcher may want to learn the psychological characteristics of the decision; the ultimate purpose might be to change such decisions so that such patients would choose abortion. Under the Commission's recommendations and 1981 DHHS regulations, consent would apparently not be required. The study would not even be research involving human subjects if identifiers were deleted from the records. Yet some of these women who chose not to abort might well object to being an essential part of the study. Even though they have no "interests" in the study, they might still want to consent. They would not, however, have been given the information they desire in order to determine whether to be part of the study.

PUBLIC ACCESS TO MEETINGS

Finally, let us examine one last suggestion the Commission offered. This was that the DHHS consider whether or not there is a right of public access to IRB meetings and to the records of IRBs. While the Commission admitted that the legal right of public access is controversial and unsettled and that it could not reach agreement on recommending that IRBs be required to meet in public, it did say it "supported the principle of open meetings."[26] Behind this is a fundamental debate over whether IRBs are governing agencies and thus subject to federal and local laws requiring open meetings, or whether they are agencies of local institutions where private meetings may be more tolerable, at least in cases where the institutions themselves are not public bodies.

The question has implications far beyond the right of the public to attend meetings and see records of the IRB. If the IRB is a governmental body, then public values expressed through the political process ought to dominate IRB decision making. This calls into question the legitimacy of committees designed to reflect only the value consensus of the institution. At least if the institution is private, the public has little justification for concern that its values be reflected in the IRB, but also has little reason to delegate to such a private group decisions about which the public has a great interest. Unfortunately the current regulations fail to discuss the issue of public access to IRB meetings. In fact, as we shall see in the next chapter, in some ways the IRB is functioning as a public agent; as such, it should be broadly representative of the public rather than the more specialized research community, which currently dominates it.

The 1981 regulations are the culmination of years of careful consideration and effort on the part of members of DHEW, the National Commission, and DHHS. We are certainly much better off with the regulations than without them. Yet, as I have argued, there is room for improvement. The following suggestions summarize the changes that I have argued merit support:

1. Regulations under DHHS jurisdiction should apply to all research involving human subjects (rather than to only research conducted or funded by the DHHS) including experiments involving minimum risk and research not funded or otherwise regulated by DHHS.

2. The DHHS should redefine "human subject" so as not to exclude persons who have died and those who are not identifiable.

3. The DHHS should maintain uniform minimal standards for expediting reviews, but these standards should be changed to include studies that are currently exempt.

4. In reviewing research, all effects including the long-term effects of

applying knowledge gained in research should be considered when assessing risks and benefits.

5. Considerations of equity should not be limited to the selection of subjects, but should extend to questions of research design and execution so that there is a fair distribution of benefits between subjects and others.

6. Consent waivers should be permitted only when there is firm evidence that it is reasonable to assume subjects would not object to having information withheld (or in exceptional cases when subjects are conscripted following due process).

CHAPTER SEVEN

Institutional Review Boards: Professional or Representative?

Advisory and review committees have emerged in the last decade as a major force in the scientific enterprise. Critics plead for increasingly stringent and inclusive review mechanisms while researchers see scientific progress grinding to a halt as if "someone had deliberately set out to destroy all major research efforts." Human experimentation committees, now generally referred to as institutional review boards (IRBs), constitute the most significant example. If these committees are to serve the purpose of providing adequate protection of potential research subjects while also furthering important research objectives, it is critical that there be a conscious, carefully worked out understanding of the various proposed models of IRBs so that the best alternative model may be chosen. The aim of this chapter will be to work toward achieving this end.

Since its opening, over 460 multiple assurances and over 4,750 single assurances have been filed for research involving human subjects with the National Institutes of Health, a division of the Department of Health and Human Services (DHHS), not including boards not directly related to the federal government requirements. This makes the sheer size of the movement an important case study.

A second, more theoretical feature of the committees also makes their study important. As an effort to bring interdisciplinary professionals and laypersons into the scientific advisory and review process they are an intermediate case between two models of the review committee. On the one hand is the interdisciplinary professional review model. The national technology assessment panels are examples. Recognizing that scientific policy review and technology assessment are complicated tasks requiring many skills, review committees are not limited to natural scientists. Sociologists, lawyers, clergy and professional philosophers are included.

At the other extreme is what might be called the "jury model." The jury is one of the most potent voices of the ordinary person. Its task is to reflect the common sense of the reasonable person. Expertise relevant to the case at hand is not only not necessary, it often disqualifies one from serving on the jury.

A slight variant on the jury model is what might be called the representative model. As with the jury model the representative model of committee responsibility requires no specific substantive, technical skill. It does, however, require a generalized skill not found in the jury member. The representative ought to be skilled in perceiving and communicating the views of his or her constituents.

Probably no advisory or review committee functions in the ideal type jury model, although paradoxically judicial case law, which is the source of any of the rules of review in groups like IRBs, depends directly on the jury's judgment. The community advisory boards of local hospitals approach the notion of expertise that stands behind the jury or representative models. Diverse, clearly lay representation is expected. To the extent community elections to the committees are based on any concept of expertise at all, the notion of expertise is highly generalized. Elected individuals are expected to be generally wise and skilled in communicating the community's views, not in specific substantive areas like medicine, hospital administration, or law.

IRBs at the moment stand somewhere between the two extremes of the interdisciplinary professional as model and the jury model. Over the last decade they have evolved, broadening their base of representation. Currently they are beginning to look very much like interdisciplinary groups of professionals, but there are clear signs of movement toward the jury or at least the representative model. Behind this shift stands a movement in our understanding of the nature of these committees and the kinds of problems they must solve. First, I will trace the evolution in the committee composition; then I will examine a series of conceptual problems which are linked to this shifting understanding of the committee's role. The thesis argued in this chapter is that there are presently inherent conflicts in the premises underlying IRBs. Until these are clarified and dealt with explicitly, tensions, inefficiencies, and even failures are inevitable.

1. *The Birth of Lay Authority: The Historical Context.* The entire concept of committee review of experimental protocols using human subjects is remarkably new. In part that is because the concept of the experiment in medicine and biology is uniquely modern. While trying out of new remedies was advocated in ancient medicine, the concept of systematically designing experiments for the primary purpose of gaining knowledge is a modern phenomenon. During the nineteenth century an ethic of consulting with one's colleagues evolved. Thomas Percival, whose code we have seen is the

foundation of Anglo-American medical ethics, warns of the need for collegial approval, but in a manner that noticeably disregards the need for subject consent or involvement in the review.

> Whenever cases occur, attending with circumstances not heretofore observed . . . remedies and new methods of chirurgical treatment should be devised. But in the accomplishment of the salutary purpose, the gentlemen of the faculty should be scrupulously and conscientiously governed by sound reason, just analogy, or well authenticated facts. And no such trials should be instituted without a previous consultation of the physicians or surgeons according to the nature of the case.[1]

This vague commitment to one's colleagues to justify experimental treatment was all that existed of peer review until well into the twentieth century. The Nuremberg Code and the major professional medical codes (such as the A.M.A. Code, the World Medical Association's Declaration of Helsinki, and the British Medical Association's policy on experimental research on human beings) say nothing about committee or other peer review.

In 1953 with the opening of the National Institutes of Health Clinical Center the federal government had to face the question of experimentation ethics directly. On November 17, NIH issued a set of guidelines referred to as "Group Consideration of Clinical Research Procedures Deviating From Accepted Medical Practice or Involving Unusual Hazard."[2] The guidelines applied only to intramural research at NIH where a medical review committee reviewed studies involving ethical considerations.[3] The primary responsibility for the ethics of research was, however, placed on the individual investigator. Written consent from the subject was required where there was the possibility of an unusual hazard. At NIH panels passed judgment on the relative scientific merit of the proposals for extramural research and the Advisory Councils of the respective Institutes eventually evaluated wider social considerations. The panels were thought to be performing a scientific task—the determining of scientific merit. The Advisory Councils, more diverse in their backgrounds, were the first channel for interdisciplinary or more lay review. Even here, however, there was no explicit requirement to employ any particular ethical principles or guidelines in the evaluation.

In 1962 the Law-Medicine Research Institute of Boston University conducted a survey of eighty-six departments of medicine. In fifty-two responses they found only nine institutions that had procedural documents for experimentation committees, although twenty-two departments had committees examining the questions concerning the use of human subjects.[4] William Curran, Institute Director in 1962, concludes that at this time there was a general skepticism toward ethical guidelines and sets of procedures concerning the conduct of research. Researchers were to be guided "by their own professional judgment and controlled by their own ethical standards as well as those of their institution."[5]

Up to this point the struggle was framed in terms of the investigator having the primary obligation for review. The newer idea of review by a committee of the investigator's peers was a secondary consideration. By 1964 a group headed by Robert Livingston, then Associate Chief for Program Development of the Division of Research at NIH, had been formed to clarify the government's ethical and legal obligations for research review. They concluded, among other things, that "a professional group should be encouraged to formulate a statement of principles relating to the moral and ethical aspects of clinical investigation."[6] A consensus was emerging that gave the biomedical community as a professional group the responsibility for monitoring the ethics of its research. But the response of James A. Shannon, the Director of NIH from 1955 until 1968, contained within it the seeds for a new round in the debate—the continued broadening of the review mechanisms to include the views of other professionals and of "our society at large." According to Shannon:

> The problem is to conceive of a manner by which the statement of principles will be assured of endorsement as a consensus position which can serve as a positive guide to the conduct of clinical research. The advisors recommend that this statement of principles be developed by an appropriate professional group. We are inclined to think a broader approach may be necessary.
>
> To win general acceptance within not only the medical research community but also our society at large, the final statement of principles should probably emerge from a group which includes representatives of the whole ethical, moral and legal interests of society. The nature of this group and the manner of its convening remains the critical question in acting upon recommendation number one.[7]

This profound insight projected the evolution of the layperson's role in experimentation review over the next decade up to the present. Beginning in 1965 some form of committee review was required for all investigation involving human subjects supported by the Public Health Service. Revisions in NIH guidelines of other governmental action since then have regularly broadened the representation on the committee.

The National Advisory Health Council on December 3, 1965, passed the first resolution officially mandating committee review.

> Be it resolved that the National Advisory Health Council believes that Public Health Service support of clinical research and investigation involving human beings should be provided only if the judgment of the investigator is subject to prior review by his institutional associates to assure an independent determination of the protection of the rights and welfare of the individual or individuals involved, of the appropriateness of the methods used to secure informed consent, and of the risks and potential medical benefits of the investigation.[8]

The February 8, 1966, policy statement of the Surgeon General required prior review of the judgment of the principal investigator or program director by "a committee of his institutional associates" which was to be filed with the grant application. The July 1, 1966, revision provided more details for the institutional review. "The institution shall be responsible for developing the administrative mechanism for review, surveillance, and advice." The Public Health Service required explicitly that the review assure an independent determination of: (1) the rights and welfare of the individual or individuals, (2) the appropriateness of the methods used to secure informed consent, and (3) the risks and potential medical benefits of the investigation. It also required that the committee of associates have no vested interest in the specific project involved.

The instructions on the makeup of the committee, however, were extremely vague. The institution could utilize staff, consultants, or both, and the policy recognized that "any group responsible for review should possess not only specific competence to comprehend the scientific content of the investigations reviewed, but also other competencies pertinent to the judgments that need to be made." The interdisciplinary model of committee review was well on its way to establishment. Each institution was required to file assurances with the Public Health Service including a report of "the competencies represented in the committees of associates utilized for review." Shannon's proleptic sense that the perspectives of the society at large had to be included in committees dealing with experimentation review is lost. The concept is one of peer review, but peer is taken narrowly as peers of the researcher, never as peers of the subject or as the reasonable citizen implied in the phrase "jury of one's peers." The committee is explicitly a group of "associates of the investigator."

On May 1, 1969, a revision of the 1966 guidelines introduced substantive and procedural changes.[9] The peer group of the researcher's associates slides almost imperceptibly in the direction of a broader group. The space devoted to committee makeup reflects greater awareness that a narrow group of biomedical scientists would be inadequate for the job. It was now mandated that "the committee must be composed of sufficient members with varying backgrounds to assure complete and adequate review. . . ." The guidelines go on to require that "the membership should possess not only broad specific competence to comprehend the nature of the research, but also other competencies necessary in the judgment as to acceptability of the research in terms of institutional regulations, relevant law, standards of professional practice, and community acceptance." Most of these specifications fit nicely into the interdisciplinary professional model. Competencies including "position, earned degrees, board certifications, licensures, memberships, and other indications of experience and competence" had to be identified in the assurance filed with the Public Health Service—obvious traditional measures of professional standing. But skill in judging "community acceptance" had crept onto the list for the first time—a skill not normally measured by board certifications or licensure. Both ability to judge the project in terms of "community attitudes" as well as indicating the various competencies of board members mentioned above remain included in the 1981 regulations, which are in effect as of this publication.[10]

At the end of 1971 a revision of the 1969 DHEW policy on the protection of human subjects appeared. The famous yellow booklet had requirements for committees made up essentially similar to the 1969 guidelines. On May 30, 1974, DHEW issued regulations, revising the guidelines that had been in effect since December, 1971. One change was that the latter guidelines state that no fewer than five persons are required to be on the committee[11] while the earlier guidelines required only that the committee be composed of "sufficient members."[12] The new 1981 regulations maintain the requirement of at least five members.

Another concern since the 1974 regulations is that there be at least one member of the committee who is not affiliated with the research organization apart from their committee membership.[13] This requirement is maintained in the 1981 regulations.[14]

Another change that has come about is the requirement that the committee members have sufficiently diverse backgrounds. The 1971 requirements stated:

> In addition to possessing the professional competence to review specific activities, the committee should be able to determine acceptability of the proposal in terms of institutional commitments and regulations, applicable law, standards of professional conduct and practice and community attitudes. The committee *may* therefore need to include persons whose primary concerns lie in these areas rather than in the conduct of research, development, and service programs of the types supported by the DHEW.[15]

The 1974 regulations were revised to make the requirement that the committee be composed of varying professions mandatory, rather than optional. The 1974 regulations stated the committee "must" include persons concerned in the areas such as applicable law, standards of professional conduct and practice, and community attitudes.[16] They stated "no committee shall consist entirely of members of a single professional group."[17] The regulations, however, did not state any precise number of how many such members should make up the committee. Following this the National Commission had suggested in its comments on recommendation three (A) that, in order to assure that the committee as a whole has both sufficient numbers of individuals with "scientific competence necessary to analyze accurately and thoroughly the risks and benefits" as well as "persons who are familiar with the ethical issues in research" that "at least one-third but no more than two-thirds of the IRB members should be scientists. . . ."[18] (The merits of the Commission taking the view that determining the risks and the benefits is a job best reserved for scientists will be considered shortly.) The Commission's notion that special care should be taken to assure that committees are sufficiently diverse is an important one. Unfortunately, however, the 1981 regulations do not incorporate any quota as was suggested by the Commission. All that is required is that each IRB must include at least one member whose primary concerns are in non-scientific areas such as lawyers, ethicists, and members of the clergy.[19]

The 1981 recommendations did, however, include a rule ensuring fair representation of each gender by stating that no committee may consist entirely of either sex. This rule had been suggested in the Commission's earlier work, but had been phrased less clearly.[20] This requirement seems to be the result of the concern that lay representation be sufficient since obviously this requirement would have no relevance to professional competence.

Another change appearing in the 1981 regulations—which were a response to the National Commission's suggestion to do so[21]—is the additional statement that

> If an IRB regularly reviews research that involves a vulnerable category of subjects, including but not limited to subjects covered by other subparts of this part, the IRB shall include one or more individuals who are primarily concerned with the welfare of these subjects.[22]

This statement seems to open the door further to encouraging lay participation, although of course it is also possible that particular professionals may also at times meet the requirement of having a special interest in the welfare of specific subject populations.

2. *Theory and Structure of the Experimentation Committee.* We have no explicit theory of what these committees are supposed to be able to do, of what purposes they are to serve, of what skills their members ought to have. While we are beginning to develop a serious literature on the substantive issues of experimentation ethics, no one has stopped to ask what specifically it is that the committee is supposed to do. In part this results from a lack of understanding of what the committees, in fact, do. At least two excellent sociological studies of committee functioning are now available from Bernard Barber and his colleagues, and from Bradford Gray.

It is not my objective to add to these empirical descriptions of committee workings. Rather I want to draw from these existing studies, from my own experience as a member of two busy committees and chairman of a less active one, and from general, informal knowledge of the workings of several other committees, in an attempt to set out some of the theoretical problems of committee purpose and function. I will conclude that the ambiguities are so great that, until the theory of the committee is clarified and appropriate structural changes are made in accord with that theory, it is impossible for the experimentation committee to successfully fulfill its tasks.

I am not going to argue that the committee members are irresponsible, that they are not dedicated in their roles. I have, on the contrary, been generally highly impressed with the quality of commitment and the willingness of committee members to ask tough questions, sometimes of their own colleagues. Furthermore, I am convinced that the present committee mechanisms function to protect human subjects far better than the reliance on the investigator's personal judgments which dominated a decade ago. My concern is principally with a clearer definition of what the committee ought to be and, derivatively, what its makeup ought to be, if it is to fulfill its tasks.

A. GENERAL PURPOSES

At the most general level the purposes of the experimentation committee are fairly clear. The task is to protect human subjects from possible harms and wrongs that they might suffer during the course of biomedical and now behavioral research. It does this by assuring that the risks to subjects are reasonable in relation to anticipated benefits, if any, to subjects and the importance of the knowledge that may reasonably be expected to result, by assuring adequately informed consent, protection of privacy, equitable subject selection, and so forth.

We have seen, in the last chapter, that there are some inconsistencies when the DHHS on the one hand uses the committee structure to accomplish these important objectives while at the same time it does not require that *all* research using humans be subject to IRB review. In spite of such inconsistencies, however, the general objectives of the committees are reasonably well defined. What skills are necessary in order to assess risks and welfare, to determine what information is necessary for an adequately informed consent, and to project risks and benefits to the subject and society?

B. SKILLS FOR RESPONSIBLE COMMITTEE REVIEW

While guidelines for committee selection speak freely of necessary competencies, experience, and maturity, no one seems to have given serious attention to exactly what these might be. If it is true that the IRB is an ambiguous case somewhere between the interdisciplinary professional model and the more representative model, we would expect both kinds of skills to be necessary.

1. *Professional Skills.* From the beginning the committees have done a decent job of accumulating a group with knowledge of the science involved in the research. The committee must judge the benefits of the research, its scientific merit, how much will be learned, and what specific harms might come to the subjects. This is the kind of skill one would expect from a committee set up as a group of the researcher's "institutional associates." His peers should be capable of contributing these skills. Barber found that in four-fifths of the institutions in his study, most of the committee members came from the highest levels including clinical, administrative, and academic hierarchies. At others, the majority came from the intermediate level, but nowhere was the majority from the lower levels of the professional hierarchy.[23]

It is now also recognized that other, non-medical professional skills are essential. There must be knowledge of the law, social science, psychology, and religious traditions if judgments about informed consent, psychological benefits and risks, and rights of subjects are to be made. Knowledge of and ability to analyze the language and structure of arguments has led to adding philosophers to committees as an essential component. Even so, Barber's group found relatively small numbers of these professionals: From personnel within the institution, eighteen percent of the committees had nurses, nine percent lawyers, another nine percent had members of the board and behavioral scientists. From outside the institution four percent had lawyers, five percent behavioral scientists; and four percent clergymen. One institution had a patient representative.[24] It seems likely that members with these non-medical professional skills will remain in a minority of many committees. This, I will argue later, raises some important theoretical problems about the committee's willingness to take risks.

It seems to me that possession of all of these professional skills is essential for the committee to function according to its present mandate. It is naive to believe that laymen can pick up value-relevant scientific facts without professional assistance. Recent studies reported in a professional journal or at a scientific meeting may make the research redundant. Tests may have predictable side effects anticipated only by those knowing in detail the methods used. A new legal decision across the country may place the committee and the researchers in jeopardy if a protocol is approved. Psychological harm may go quite unnoticed to the untrained eye. All of this makes these professional inputs essential.

2. *Representative or Jury Skills*. The recent recognition that the committees must also have the ability to judge community attitudes, community acceptance, and what the reasonable patient/subject would want to know about the research has complicated the skill requirements tremendously. One particular group of legal decisions involving informed consent makes clear that a radically different set of talents must be present in the committee. Beginning in California in 1969 and more frequently since then, the courts have broken precedent in a series of cases involving arguments about informed consent.[25] While the specifics of the cases vary tremendously, the principle involved is similar and is terribly important for experimentation committees. The cases all involve arguments that some patient or subject has not been given adequate information upon which to base his consent for research or treatment. The defense used by the medical profession in these cases has been the standard one. The professional argues that his colleagues hold a consensus that the particular piece of information ought not to have been transmitted. It was thought too trivial or too disturbing to the patient or subject. It was either in the patient's interests that he not be told, or more ordinarily, simply such a small risk that the professionals agree that the layman should not be troubled with it. Until recently that was an adequate defense—provided the professional could prove (through testimony) that his

colleagues agreed with his judgment that the piece of information was not necessary for an adequately informed consent.

The recent decisions reject this argument on principle. Whether or not the reasonable person would want to know something is logically still an open question even if there is a consensus among the professional group that they do not think the layperson ought to know it. Judging whether the information is to be transmitted is fundamentally not a technical judgment according to these recent decisions. It is something the reasonable person can judge for himself or herself. The legal opinions have also unanimously pointed to the conclusion that even if professionals agree that the information is not required for an adequately informed consent, the reasonable person—as measured by the opinion of a jury—can still decide that it is required.

The principle of the reasonable person as the proper judge of what is required for an informed consent and the claim that a professional consensus is not an adequate measure of what the reasonable person would want to know have crucial significance for the functioning of the IRB. Professionals are by definition a special class with a special perspective on critical issues in the experimentation situation. As such they are particularly lacking in competence in judging what the reasonable layperson would want to know for his or her consent to be informed. Professionals are unique not only in their socioeconomic status and their ethnic and sex group, but more critically in their occupation. Medical researchers, by definition, have a unique commitment to the value of research. If they are asked to evaluate the relative harms to the subject in comparison to the benefits to be gained by society from the pursuit of knowledge, they cannot avoid incorporating their conviction that scientific knowledge is valuable.

The problem is not simply one of cronyism. Biases created by the necessity of evaluating the research of one's personal friends and colleagues (occasionally of committee members themselves) produce some difficulties, but, in my opinion, those difficulties are not nearly as critical as the ones created by unique values held in common among a group of professionals committed to common ends—such as the pursuit of knowledge. Obviously the American Civil Liberties Union member, the construction worker, the welfare rights organizer, or the housewife would have very different instincts, but these people—the ones who might serve on a jury to determine reasonableness of the information given for informed consent—very rarely get to serve on experimentation committees. It is the task of the committee to determine how to trade off the welfare and rights of the subject against the benefits to the subject and to society, and to determine how much information is necessary for an informed consent. The determination must logically be influenced by the makeup of the committee. The absence of these "jury" or "representative" skills must influence the outcome of the review. For jury or representative skills the subject would be much better served—at least in theory—by a committee of peers of the subject rather than peers of the researcher.

C. IMPLICATIONS FOR COMMITTEE THEORY

Here then is the dilemma of the IRB: Both the professional skills and the representative or jury skills are essential, yet the two are mutually exclusive. Perhaps by chance some proper combination of professions will be able to represent the views of the reasonable person—that would be fortuitous, but unlikely. Even if that were possible, the egalitarianism and dignity of the layperson would be challenged by the professionalization of the reasonable person. It is a conclusion which saddens me, for practical solutions to the dilemma will be difficult and perhaps sometimes impossible but I believe it an inevitable conclusion which follows logically from the analysis. As one who believes fervently in the good which can come from biomedical and behavioral research, I do not want to see it mired in the continual struggle over an acceptable mechanism for review. But compromises will probably not resolve the dilemma. The theoretical implications are great. A few will be outlined.

1. The Impossibility of Neutralizing Systematic Bias. Recognizing that biomedical scientists have special perspectives, recent mandates for committees have attempted to neutralize bias by adding representatives of other professional disciplines, or even of patient and community groups. The scientist has long recognized that biases are of two types: random and systematic. The professional committee—even in its older, narrower form that included only biomedical scientists—does an excellent job of eliminating random bias. The success-driven researcher with a warped moral perspective is held in check by colleagues with more balanced perspectives. But the systematic value perspectives of the professional group (the use of scientific models, the love of rationality, and most important, the quest for knowledge and scientific progress—these values which all scientists ought to share) in principle cannot be eliminated by the establishment of a committee of those who hold those unique values. What is more, while the addition of other professional groups may eliminate the peculiar scientific value patterns, it almost certainly does not eliminate the wider constellation of values held by the educated, professional class as a whole. Even adding patient or community representatives will only dilute these systematic biases, not eliminate them. As long as one professional is on the "jury," the panel will be skewed from the view of the reasonable layperson.

2. Risk Shift and Its Implications for Experimentation Committees. An interesting phenomenon has been discovered in social psychology research in the last decade that has great potential significance for the experimentation committee. Stoner discovered that the process of decision making by committee in and of itself had a measurable impact on the decision.[26] His initial work led to the conclusion that committees as a whole reach decisions that permit more risky choices than the average of the individual views of the members of the committee would suggest. If this is the case among human experimentation committees, then the committee designed to protect subjects from extravagant risks undertaken by individual researchers will, in fact, be institutionalizing a decision-making mechanism that systematically increases the willingness to take risks on behalf of the subject. The risk-shift, as the phenomenon has been called, would, of course, still place limits on the most wild, individual risk-takers, but on average, the committee would systemically shift the judgment in favor of taking risks on behalf of the subjects.

There are several theories of why this takes place. One plausible explanation is that many committees have more high-risk takers than low-risk takers. Since, if each were to speak his or her mind, more high-risk taking opinions and arguments would be voiced, then everyone on the committee would shift somewhat in the risk-taking direction. This hypothesis has been tested by forming committees dominated by minimal-risk people, and the predicted anti-risk shift took place.[27]

The implications for experimentation committees are tremendous. If the committee includes a scientist, a clergyman, and maybe a representative of the community as anti-risk takers, in all likelihood they will stand in the minority. Even a feisty member of such a minority will find it extremely difficult to withstand the psychological pressure to cooperate in forming a consensus.

For the normal committee, however, the dominance of the committee by scientific professionals would produce the risk-shift in the direction of the researchers' values—normally in favor of the research. That is not to suggest that the scientific members of the committee are manipulative or even that they fail to exercise utmost caution in attempting to protect subjects and serve their interests—it is simply the nature of the group process. Even if it were the case that those with representative skills stood in the majority and a shift in the committee took place in the direction of those selected to serve as the peers of the subject, the consensus would still be influenced or moderated by the other perspective, thus supporting more risk than those with representative skills were willing to take.

3. *Judgments of Scientific Merit.* One of the tasks most often thought to require professional, scientific competence is the judgment of scientific merit of the proposal. Some have even proposed division of labor with one committee made up of scientists to judge the scientific merit of the proposal and another, more interdisciplinary or lay, to judge the ethical dimensions. Even here, however, if this analysis is correct, the matter is much more complicated. Merit is an ethical, or at least a value, word. We should be aroused when it is suggested that such value judgments can be made scientifically. We should separate two tasks. First, the protocol must be reviewed to see whether the results sought can theoretically be obtained by the methods, sampling, and design proposed. It seems that evaluation can be most competently carried out by scientists. Second, however, is the task of deciding how valuable the findings would be if the research is worthwhile (another value term). This second judgment will require insight into the

possible future uses of the research, which may require great scientific skills, but in the end judgments of worthiness are not scientific. Even the pure science argument that accumulation of knowledge for its own sake with nothing more than a theoretical faith that something good may come out of it justifies the research, is a non-scientific value argument. If risks to subjects are to be evaluated in part in terms of the value of the knowledge to be gained, then certainly the reasonable person's judgment must be the standard-enterprise—unless scientists are used as subjects.

There are also certainly administrative implications of the dilemma posed by the conflicting tasks of the experimentation committee.

D. ADMINISTRATIVE IMPLICATIONS

If it is the case that different committee compositions will equip the committee to serve different tasks, but that no one composition can permit it to do all its tasks well, then we should look at how committee administration has an impact on these committee functions.

1. Who Selects the Committee? None of the guidelines or regulations governing experimentation committees address themselves to the crucial question of how the committees will be selected. Selection is to be handled at the local level. Normally the head of the institution or the department appoints the committee as is the case for most academic and institutional committees. Once appointed, the chairman may have de facto power to appoint new members. He or she may nominate or simply suggest to the head of the institution new members for the committee as old members drop off, or as new government policies require new membership categories.

I have not heard any serious criticism of this mechanism of appointment. Nevertheless, there would seem to be no conceivable justification for this procedure except on the professional model or on some notion of private enterprise control of one's own institutional review mechanisms. The institution head or committee chairperson will inevitably select compatible people for the committee. Once one recognizes that there are different perspectives that will invariably be brought into the decision-making process, no matter how committed the members are to fairness, the mechanism of committee appointment must be critical. The representative or jury models would presumably depend on election or selection outside of professional channels. Community advisory boards might take over the appointment responsibility or serve as the experimentation review committee themselves. If the community board or the jury selection mechanism were used, substantial training would be required. The "grand jury" with long tenure might be the appropriate analogy. No one, to my knowledge, is addressing the question.

2. Term and Tenure. Closely related to the power of appointment is the term of office and tenure. Remarkably few committees have a formal policy on the term of office or on the power to remove someone from the committee. Since most groups appear to work in a collegial context where a close working relationship is important, formal power to fire may not be as important as the more subtle psychological pressures, on the one hand, to cooperate with the group maintaining proper group relations and, on the other, to resign if one is "incompatible." Resignations in protest have been considered by dissenting members (either those favoring more constraint on research or those objecting to too much constraint) who discover that they have slipped through the collegial net, but then they realize that to resign is to remove a dissenting voice from the committee. Under the professional model it would appear that those who are responsible for professional competence—department or institution heads—ought to have the authority to remove committee members. Under the representative model, however, the more public charges of inadequacy of representation would be the logical grounds for removal and more public mechanisms would seem appropriate.

3. *The Committee Vote.* The method of voting is logically related to the more theoretical issues we have raised. If there is a diversity of functions being served by the different members of the committee, a case can be made for the unanimous voting procedure. Any one professional competence or skill in communicating community attitudes should be sufficient to introduce a decisive objection which the other committee members would not have adequate competence to refute. If the jury model is operating, unanimous vote might be required for different reasons: The jury requires overwhelming evidence. If, by analogy, we believe that there must be overwhelming evidence that the subject will not have his rights, welfare, or other interests jeopardized before we permit him to be exposed to risks for him personally, then we may also insist on unanimity here. If the representative model variant is used and the entire committee is representing community standards, then maybe a majority or two-thirds vote would be sufficient. The same might be true if the committee represented only one professional competence. The 1981 regulations require that in order for research to be approved, a majority vote must be reached. Further, save for expedited review, voting can take place only at meetings at which a majority of the members of the IRB are present, "including at least one member whose primary concerns are in non-scientific areas."[28] This seems to assume the professional representative model to be valid.

4. *Institutional vs. Non-Institutional Membership.* The difference between institutional and non-institutional employees on the committee has recently been introduced as a way of increasing the diversity of the committee perspectives. This is independent of the professional/lay dichotomy. Whether an interdisciplinary professional model or a jury model is the basis for the committee, there would appear to be solid grounds for increasing the non-institutional representation, in order to increase the number of perspectives. If that is the case, however, the question of compensation for the non-institutional members of the committee becomes important. The principle of equal pay for equal work is important for two reasons: to secure the necessary commitment from the non-institutional members to do the work done by

institution members on company time, and to convey the fact that the non-professionals (who are likely not to be institution employees) are at least as qualified as the professionals in performing the task of the committee.

It is remarkable that there has been so little attention given to these administrative details of local human-experimentation committees. It seems clear that the administrative questions are closely linked to the more theoretical questions of committee function that I have raised. It is to be hoped that as we gain a greater understanding of what the committee ought to be doing and what skills are necessary, we will also develop more clearly formulated administrative procedures based on our theory of the experimentation committee.

CONCLUSIONS

The human experimentation committee is a fascinating case of an interdisciplinary or lay policy committee in the biomedical enterprise. Unlike both the national technology assessment panels and the community hospital advisory boards, the experimentation committees are clearly more than advisory groups. They have the power to approve or block research. They stand midway between the other two committees on the dimension of whether the committee is an interdisciplinary professional group or a lay group qualified because of the degree to which they represent community attitudes or the "reasonable person."

I have tried to show that both models are important to the experimentation committee and we have not adequately understood how the two tasks are related. I am more and more convinced that the real conflict is not between the scientific committees, which are made up of peers of the researcher (committees of associates) on the one hand, and the broader interdisciplinary professional groups on the other, but rather between the committees made up of professionals (including interdisciplinary professional committees) and those that are truly lay committees chosen because they are either typical reasonable people or because they have skills to represent the typical person.

It appears to me that the trend is clearly in the direction of a broader, more lay membership of these committees. The informed-consent court cases require that the committee be skilled in understanding the reasonable person's perspective. The courts tell us that professionals—at least medical professionals—cannot be presumed to have that perspective.

The move toward committees of half scientists and half laypeople and other professionals is part of this trend, but that cannot be the answer. The consensus of that group in principle cannot approximate the community judgment (unless one hypothesizes that the different professional groups counterbalance one another—and that seems unlikely). Even a committee of half professionals and half laypersons would not meet the objections of the representative or jury model. Two solutions seem possible.

First, the task of experimentation review could be turned over to a group more skilled in representing the community attitudes or the views of the reasonable person. At the moment, the most obvious candidate is the community hospital advisory board in institutions that have such boards. They have been elected or selected for their capacity to represent the layperson, the consumer of the hospital's services. Why these boards have not played a larger role in experimentation review is not clear to me. Certainly if they were to take on this task they would have to be provided with a supporting staff capable of providing the professional skills obviously needed and now obtained through the interdisciplinary professional group.

Second, we might have to resort to dual committees. One would be made up of professionals charged with the professional tasks of determining scientific feasibility and also judging ethical acceptability from their perspective in terms of risks and benefits, informed consent, and the knowledge to be gained. We would not expect that committee to hand down judgments to reflect the reasonable person's standards, but they would provide for the introduction of the professional skills, including judgments of risks knowable only to one with the appropriate training. The second committee would be the community committee, which would have to have, as before, adequate professional staff and would make value judgments of scientific worthiness as well as the more obviously ethical judgments.

I am inclined to think that this is a more practical, fail-safe solution. Exactly what these committees will look like must depend upon our understanding of a theory of their function and structure. It seems to me that we must continue to move in the direction of making the reasonable person the foundation of these committees in what I have called the jury, or representative, model. The professional skills must remain necessary, but the newer skills must be added. I am convinced that resolving this dilemma of providing essential but mutually exclusive skills is both difficult and necessary.

CHAPTER EIGHT

Liability and the IRB Member: The Ethical Aspects

The idea that IRB members might be personally liable for their actions while serving in an official capacity is disturbing. Equally troublesome, however, is the possibility that they could be totally immune from responsibility. In addition to the legal facts of tort liability, which have been addressed elsewhere,[1] there are also significant ethical dimensions to this question.

Certainly there are many opportunities for IRB members to make mistakes. For example, each member is responsible for assessing whether legally effective informed consent will be obtained in any protocol reviewed. It is now becoming clear (and the National Commission for the Protection of Human Subjects has affirmed) that subjects must be given information that they may reasonably be expected to desire in considering whether or not to participate in the research.[2]

Furthermore, this "reasonable subject" standard clearly leaves open the possibility that what reasonable subjects may want to know (or find material) before making a judgment to participate may be different from what reasonable IRB members think these subjects would want to know. To the extent that IRB members differ in any way from the subjects in this assessment, they may make systematic mistakes in carrying out their functions. Sooner or later some subject is going to argue—and perhaps in court—that even though the researchers and the IRB decided that he or she would not want a particular piece of information, that information was in fact precisely what the subject wanted to know. For example, researchers on an IRB might all agree that donors to a blood bank would not want to be told that the blood might be used for research. It is still very much an open question whether reasonable subjects would find that information material in deciding whether to donate blood. IRB members might be liable, legally or ethically, if they cannot demonstrate a good-faith effort to show that they attempted to determine whether subjects would really want to know the information.

As Angela Holder points out in her article "Liability and the IRB Member: The Legal Aspects," though it is possible that an institution as a corporate entity can be liable for negligent approval of a research protocol, an individual member of an IRB would not be held personally liable for the payment of any money damages.[3] Her analysis differs from that of the National Commission's view that "IRB members may be personally liable to subjects and investigators for 'malpractice' or negligence in discharging their IRB functions."[4] Besides the question of legal liability, however, policy makers and IRB members need to determine whether the law is justified or unjustified in this regard.

ARGUMENTS CONCERNING PROTECTION

The arguments favoring protection of IRB members from personal liability are obvious. Members of IRBs normally take on enormous burdens with little or no compensation, little professional reward, and often at great personal inconvenience and stress. In doing so, they are serving the long-term interests of both researchers and society. If IRB members are to do their job well, they should be encouraged to act freely without fear of personal liability. In short, the long-term greater good is served if individual members are protected.

On the other hand, so a counterargument goes, if individual IRB members are personally liable, they will be more careful in their work and take greater personal responsibility to prevent any wrongs. The issue is really an empirical one. Would greater good be served in the long run if individual members were liable or not?

Added to this argument from consequences is another related argument. If members of IRBs take on this responsibility, they deserve protection simply as a measure of compensation for the service rendered. Independent of whether this protection enables them to do a better job and therefore to serve social interests better, they might be said to have a right to be protected against personal liability.

But the notion of personal rights suggests some other ethical counterarguments. In fact the debate over whether IRB members should be personally liable for their actions in a way recapitulates the more general ethical tension that permeates IRB activity. That tension is not really between the task of serving the interests of the individual and serving the interests of society. It is, as the current DHHS regulations suggest, between one responsibility of assuring that the total benefits of the research justify the risks and another responsibility of assuring that the rights of the subject are adequately protected.[5] Doing what will produce the most benefits will not necessarily also protect the rights of the individual subjects.

This tension has radical implications for IRBs. In the general work of the

IRB it means that in reviewing protocols, judgments about protecting rights (the right to confidentiality, the right to consent) are independent of judgments about benefits and harms. For the more narrow problem of personal liability it means that individual members cannot justifiably be shielded from liability—even if it would serve long-term social interests—if that protection would violate important individual rights. Ought there be such a right to redress when the actions of IRB members violate the rights of subjects or researchers or anyone else? Do we want IRB members to act without any responsibility for their actions? The right of redress for subjects or researchers may lead to the policy conclusion that IRB members cannot be totally immune from liability.

TWO PRINCIPLES FOR A POLICY

In considering what ethical principles might be used to formulate a policy on protecting individual members from liability, two principles come immediately to mind.

The first is the principle of responsibility. The argument from responsibility assumes that individuals are in some way responsible for their actions and should be called to account when they do harm to others or violate their rights. This implies that individual IRB members should not be personally liable for harms or violations of rights *beyond* their responsibility. If we separate negligent and non-negligent actions, most IRB members ought to be personally responsible for negligence according to this view.

Of course, we may want to adopt a policy that would permit compensation to researchers or subjects regardless of whether the harm results from the IRB's negligence or not. Institutional or governmental insurance granting such recovery may be in order for harms resulting from IRB actions just as it is being proposed for harms resulting from the research. Such insurance would leave for further discussion the question of whether IRB members should be personally responsible for reimbursing the insurance fund in cases where they are negligent.

Second, we might apply the principle of equal protection. If there are protections developed for individual IRB members for any of the reasons discussed here, the protections ought to apply equally to all IRB members.

Insurance that protected physician members but not non-physician members would be unacceptable if one adopted this principle. Similarly, protections that extended to members on the payroll of the institution, but not to those outside the institution, would violate this principle. In fact, since individuals who are outside the institution are being added to IRBs because a variety of points of view is considered crucial to adequate review, those members are especially deserving of protection. As a member of an IRB not on the institution's payroll, I find that argument particularly persuasive.

The National Commission's warning on liability of IRB members should alert IRBs to take the problem seriously.[6] It seems likely that great social good would come from granting protection. But it is also clear from the mandate IRBs have been given that serving the general welfare cannot be the only basis for judgment. The rights of researchers and the rights of subjects are crucial moral factors in this enterprise as well.

PART
IV

Problems of Research Design and Subject Recruitment

CHAPTER NINE

Justice and the Semi-Randomized Clinical Trial

If the three principles developed in Part II are to be the core of an ethic for research involving human subjects in which the subject is a partner in the research, a number of important implications follow for the design of research and the recruitment of subjects. In this and the other chapters in Part IV, some of these implications will be explored. One complicated example of a problem arises when subjects have a strong preference for one treatment arm in a randomized clinical trial. The problem is even more complex if the subjects are so poorly off that, for purposes of consideration of the principle of justice, they can be considered among the least well-off of the population. In such circumstances researchers working with subjects may have to shift to what I shall call a "semi-randomized clinical trial."

Consider a typical study on a chronically ill patient with a terminal illness such as cancer. To what extent does justice require that subjects in the typical oncology protocol have access to whichever treatment arm they prefer? Should an IRB insist, contrary to common practice and FDA regulation, that oncology patients be allowed to receive the experimental compound in a clinical trial if the subjects are convinced they would be better off receiving it? The argument favoring this policy would be that the oncology patient who is a member of a least well-off group (compared with others who might be touched by the protocol) should have his or her judgment on available treatment respected since this would predictably improve the lot of a least well-off person. Justice, therefore, would require this policy.

I assume that most persons find this implication absurd. Most will

The author is grateful to Robert J. Levine and Emil Freireich for helpful comments on an earlier draft of this paper.

probably find the subject's action irrational. The modification is at least contrary to standard research practice and thought to be potentially damaging to good research. The argument is that such choice is irrational on the part of the subject since research cannot morally be conducted unless there is a legitimate scientific doubt about which of two (or more) treatment options is in the patient's interest. Patients thus have no basis for preferring the experimental treatment. Should they prefer it, they then have been misled by the hope for success.

I am convinced this argument is erroneous. For a protocol to be justified there must be legitimate scientific doubt about which option is medically preferable. It does not follow, though, that individual patients may not have legitimate idiosyncratic, perhaps psychological, reasons for preferring one arm of the study over the other. Some individuals are conservative in their biases and would prefer not to participate in research until the intervention in question is tested further. We recognize the right of such patients to refuse to participate in the study, in effect acting on their conservative world view. Other pateints may have uniquely interventionistic world views. They take the view that when in doubt, they should gamble with the high-risk high-gain option. There is nothing irrational about patients, based on their unique psychological world views, preferring one treatment arm over another in spite of the fact that there is no objective *medical* difference known to exist between them. Right now the conservative least well-off patient has the right to withdraw from the study and get the standard treatment, but the interventionistic patient does not have the right to withdraw and get the experimental treatment. If such a patient may rationally prefer that course, justice requires that he be given that opportunity.

I propose that we consider a "semi-randomized clinical trial." Before I discuss its merits, it will be useful to review the ways it differs from the traditional trial. This latter trial begins with a sample whose members are asked to consent to be randomized, let us say, between control or standard treatment and experimental treatment. Some in the sample drop out. They receive some version of the standard treatment, but are not followed. They constitute group 1 in Figure 1. Those who consent are then randomized into the two treatment arms (groups 2a and 2b in Figure 1), and results are compared.

I propose two modifications, which will result in what I call a "semi-randomized clinical trial," in order to fulfill the requirements of justice. First, those who presently refuse randomization (group 1) should be given the option of a standardized form of the usual treatment and should be asked to consent to have their case followed as part of the study. Those who consent remain in the study as group 1b; those refusing (group 1a) are, of course, lost to the follow-up. Second, before randomization, subjects should also be given the option to drop out of the randomization, receive the experimental treatment, and be followed like the non-randomized standard treatment group. They would form a new non-randomized experimental group (group

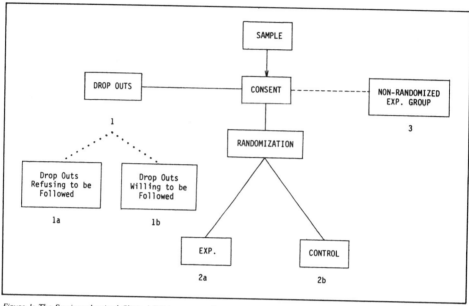

Figure 1: The Semi-randomized Clinical Trial

Reprinted From Clinical Research, Vol. 31, No. 1, February, 1983
Published by Charles B. Slack, Inc., Medical Publisher, © AFCR

3). The result will be two non-randomized groups (groups 1b and 3) and two randomized ones (groups 2a and 2b), each pair containing a standard treatment group and an experimental treatment group. The result will be that one group of least well-off patients (group 3), which is now deprived of a treatment it desires for good reason, will have an opportunity to have their interests served, thus meeting the demands of the principle of equity.

The main argument against this semi-randomized trial is a scientific one—that the sample is contaminated by the opportunity to opt for the experimental treatment without randomization. To this may be added the argument from efficiency that it will take longer to get an adequate randomized sample. It should be recognized that these are both arguments from beneficence, that is, they are arguments that less benefit will come or greater costs will be incurred if these patients are given this opportunity. As an argument from beneficence, however, it does not cut against the concern for equity or justice upon which the proposal of a semi-randomized trial is based. Just as the right of patients to consent (based on autonomy) cannot be overridden by consideration of good research design (beneficence), so the right of a least well-off group to be benefitted (based on justice) cannot be overridden on beneficence grounds.

The researcher and the IRB remain faced with the unhappy conflict between the claims of good science (beneficence) and the claims of justice. This dilemma persists unless it can be shown that the semi-randomized design turns out to be better science as well as better ethics. I think this position can be defended.

The scientific argument for use of semi-randomized design is longer and more complicated than the ethical argument, and, in the end, the claim of justice is independent of the argument about scientific validity. Here we might have just another example of what morality requires being scientifically unacceptable and what science requires being morally unacceptable.

We need to review the scientific argument for the semi-randomized trial. It is well recognized by persons sophisticated in research design that in order to generalize findings of such a randomized clinical trial to general clinical use, some critical assumptions must be made.[1] Among these is the assumption that the results obtained from a randomized experimental group (group 2a) are comparable to the ones that would be obtained from medically indentical patients who had not been randomized—patients such as those who might eventually receive the treatment in routine clinical practice. Likewise, it must be assumed that the randomized control (or standard treatment) group (group 2b) produced results that are identical to those that would be found in a non-randomized group receiving the standard treatment. While these assumptions are plausible, they are not necessarily true. In fact subtle differences among populations is the reason for adopting the randomization strategy in the first place.

It would be nice—scientifically more elegant—if we had some partial test to assess the truth of these assumptions. I therefore propose following the dropouts, creating a second control group (the non-randomized group 1b). With these two control groups (1b and 2b) one could test the hypothesis that the medical and social characteristics of those willing to be randomized (2b) and those not so willing (1b) are identical. One could also compare the results of the two groups. Additional techniques designed to test the impact of both physician and patient preferences have been suggested by Freireich.[2]

A study by the Boston Inter-Hospital Liver Group on "Therapeutic Portacaval Anastomosis" published in 1974 in *Gastroenterology* produced a startling conclusion. Patients were randomized between surgical and medical treatment options. Some patients who were randomized into the surgery group nevertheless refused the surgery. To everyone's surprise, it was found that "those patients who were selected for surgery, but who refused it, inexplicably had the best survival of any group in the study."[3]

Those who were randomized to surgery but insisted on medical treatment did better than those randomized to medical treatment. The results were replicated at two separate institutions.[4] Were no data collected on the experimental surgery group dropouts, a remarkable conclusion would have been missed. If dropouts (before and after randomization) are followed, we have the opportunity to test whether a randomized group is identical in relevant diagnostic and outcome variables to a group of non-randomized patients who choose the treatment option because they are convinced it is better for them. If the result is a difference between the randomized and non-randomized groups (for example, between 2b and 1b or between 2a and 3), we may legitimately ask if the data from the randomized group can justifiably be applied to the general population. We, of course, should not conclude that the non-randomized group is identical to the general population of potential users. If a difference in the two control groups (1b and 2b) appears, we are left with the puzzle of which is the more appropriate group for comparing to the general population.

If the randomized and non-randomized groups appear identical in composition and results, we have some tentative supportive evidence to back what otherwise is a blind assumption: that the randomized group is similar to the rest of the population. Since the non-randomized controls (1b) are there for the asking, it is hard to see why they are not followed. Good science and good ethics as well would seem to demand making the comparison.

Likewise, once the problem is realized it seems clear that good science would also require comparing a randomized experimental group (2a) to a non-randomized one (3) made up of patients who, for one reason or another, believe the experimental treatment is good for them. The results of the comparison would help support or call into question what until now is a blind, unwarranted assumption: that patients willing to be randomized who are getting the experimental treatment (2a) are in all relevant respects like the eventual patient in the general population who may receive the treatment on a non-randomized basis. The comparison at least permits us to test whether the willingness to be randomized is itself a critical variable.

The size of the non-randomized experimental group (3) may present some unexpected problems. If a large number of subjects choose the non-randomized experimental treatment, the IRB should be concerned that the initial judgments justifying randomization (that experimental and control options are similar in benefit-harm ratios) may not be warranted. If the research is legitimately undertaken only when there is real doubt on the part of the researchers which treatment is better, we can expect that most potential subjects will likewise be indifferent and therefore will not object to being randomized. In fact, they may have no basis for expressing a preference. If that is the case, our non-randomized experimental group (3) may be shockingly small. If that is the result, I am contending it may lead to worse science. The non-randomized experimental group (3) may not be large enough to test the hypothesis that it is identical to the randomized experimental group (2a). To that I would reply that ethics nevertheless requires that if no one wants to enter the non-randomized experimental group (3), then no one should have to enter it.

At the present time, a random sample is already contaminated by the requirement that patients should be permitted to drop out and receive the standard treatment. We often fail to take advantage of the valuable data the dropout could contribute. I am now arguing that giving patients the opportunity to drop out in favor of the experimental treatment would only contaminate the sample somewhat more. In the exchange we would gain two things: First we would have modified the research design so as to benefit a least well-off group. That is the important change. But second, we would gain the opportunity to test hypotheses about the contamination. We could compare randomized and non-randomized groups in a way never possible before, and we would increase our warrant for the assumption that the results of the protocol can be transferred to the general population.

FINAL TEST

Let us test the semi-randomized design against the three basic principles of ethics of the Belmont Report. First, considering respect for persons and the autonomy that demands, there can be no doubt that the semi-randomized trial enhances autonomy of subjects, compared to the forced-choice standard randomized design, where in order to get a chance at the experimental treatment patients have to agree to the coercive offer in which they will be randomized and run a risk of being placed in the control group.

The test of beneficence is ambiguous. The semi-randomized trial will require a somewhat larger sample because there is an extra experimental group. It will also require following the group presently refusing randomization and dropping out of the study. It will be seen as contaminating the sample by permitting additional dropouts. But the sample is already contaminated by the dropouts who refuse to consent to be randomized. Furthermore, as never before, the researcher has a chance to study the contamination. He or she has both experimental and control groups (3 and 1b) that are non-randomized so a direct comparison can be made. Moreover, he or she gains some preliminary evidence for what until now has been only a blind assumption about the relationship between the randomized group and the general population. On balance it is debatable whether the semi-randomized design is more beneficial than the full randomization. I am inclined to think semi-randomization is better science, but others might balance the benefits of the alternatives differently.

When the criterion of justice is added to the calculation, the result becomes lopsided in favor of semi-randomization. Now one group of least well-off patients gets to choose its preferred course by dropping out of the study and getting the standard treatment. The other group of least well-off, however, is forced into randomization with all the trauma that may involve for some who desperately want the experimental treatment. Justice—in terms of serving the interests of the least well-off—seems to come down strongly on the side of permitting this small subgroup to choose the experimental arm.

The new regulations and the Belmont Report force researchers and IRBs to move beyond autonomy (or respect for persons) and beneficence to a consideration of justice—justice in the selection of subjects and justice in designing research protocols. Justice is therefore a new item on the agenda. The implications are enormous. It will certainly mean different evaluations of protocols. It may even turn out—if I am correct—that promoting justice in this case also produces better science.

CHAPTER TEN

Subjects Who Benefit Because They Are Miserable

The principle of justice poses special problems when the target research subject group is particularly poorly off. In the last chapter this meant exploring the design of research to see if subjects could receive additional benefit by modifying the design of the research. A closely related problem arises when research is justified because it benefits least well-off groups. I have conceded that it is acceptable to target research on the least well-off in the society in cases where everyone agrees they would benefit (as, for example, in experiments with varying levels of guaranteed income).

There is, however, a special sub-group of these experiments where everyone agrees the subjects would benefit, but the only reason they would benefit from the experiment is that they are so poorly off to begin with and the benefits accompany the research (as payments or health care), but are not part of the research intervention itself. Something peculiar happens when we argue that we can target for particularly unfortunate people as subjects because they have their lot improved from the experiment, but the only reason they will improve is that they are starting so low. Recall, for example, Thomas Percival's strong defense of experimentation that it is "for the public good, and in especial degree advantageous to the poor."[1]

In recent years, the troubles of Saul Krugman and his team of researchers have recalled the Percival argument and have also clearly illustrated that research on human subjects is a social, even political, act with complex ethical ramifications. Working at the Willowbrook State School for mentally retarded children on New York's Staten Island, beginning in the 1950s, Dr. Krugman discovered that, because of poor sanitary conditions, hepatitis was endemic among the youngsters there.

To gain a better understanding of the disease and to attempt to immunize the children against it, Krugman and his team decided to inject hepatitis virus into many children as they were admitted to the institution.[2] From 1956, when the research began, until 1971, when it ended, more than 750 mentally retarded children were included in the study.

The research at Willowbrook has been attacked by a member of the Medical Committee on Human Rights, by Harvard anesthesiologist Henry Beecher, and by many others.[3] It has also been the subject of several rounds of letters published in *The Lancet*.[4] In one such letter, Stephen Goldby strongly argued against the view that performing experiments on normal or mentally retarded children when no benefit for them can result is justified.

Research on human subjects has always placed the physician-experimenter in an awkward position. We have seen that the Hippocratic oath charges the physician to do what he thinks will benefit his patient. But if we define an "experiment" as a procedure designed and carried out to gain knowledge—at least in part for the future benefit of others—then any such experiment may go beyond the immediate needs of a given patient.

THE WORLD MEDICAL ASSOCIATION'S COMMITMENT

The changing philosophy of the World Medical Association (WMA) illustrates this problem. In 1949, the WMA met in London and adopted an International Code of Medical Ethics. It said in part: "Under no circumstances is a doctor permitted to do anything that would weaken the physical or mental resistance of a human being except from strictly therapeutic or prophylactic indications imposed in the interest of his patient."[5] Some interventions performed with this as the main goal might also permit data to be gathered, but that would merely be a coincidence. Interventions unrelated to therapeutic intent would be excluded. By 1954, the WMA was becoming uncomfortable with its commitment exclusively to the individual patient. That year the organization adopted its "Principles for Those in Research and Experimentation," which, while warning that there must be "strict adherence to the general rules of respect of the individual," also explicitly recognized that experiments may be conducted on healthy subjects.[6]

By 1964, the WMA had clearly abandoned the individual patient-centered commitment of 1949 in a new set of recommendations, "because it is essential that the results of laboratory experiments be applied to human beings to further scientific knowledge and to help suffering humanity."[7]

Today, not only the regulations of the World Medical Association but those of the Nuremberg Code (as we have seen) and the United States government as well justify human experiments if, among other requirements, the risks compare favorably with the foreseeable benefits to the subject *or to others*. Hence, the Hippocratic tradition regarding human experimentation has been amended to include a concern for suffering humanity—and, of course, for scientific progress.

Yet this same commitment to benefit society may also have opened the door for the type of experimentation conducted at Willowbrook in which mentally retarded children were injected with the hepatitis virus. Experiments are justified once an experimenter can convince himself or herself that the risks are outweighed by the possible benefits, including the potential benefits to people who were not included in the experiment. Yet critics of the Willowbrook experiments charged that Krugman's application of human experimentation was an abusive subordination of an individual's rights to the interests of research for the benefit of society. When challenged, Krugman claimed that he was indeed working specifically to benefit the children upon whom he was experimenting. He made an interesting argument: Conditions at Willowbrook are miserable by any standard, and hepatitis is so widespread that the children included in the study get a *controlled* exposure to the same viral strain they would be exposed to anyway at the institution. Furthermore, the children in the study group are housed in a "special, well-equipped and well-staffed unit where they would be isolated from exposure to other infectious diseases which were prevalent in the institution—namely, shigellosis, parasitic infections, and respiratory infections."[8] At a symposium on the ethics of his research held at New York University School of Medicine, Krugman further defended his work as "beneficial for the child, because immunity would be conferred."[9] And he further argued that the Willowbrook study would one day afford protection not only to the Willowbrook children but also to their families, to employees of the school, and to worldwide populations plagued by hepatitis for many generations.[10]

But doubts remain. It is uncertain that the study was really designed to protect the Willowbrook children from illness. Further, it is uncertain that the experiments were adequately explained to parents. For example, an early version of the consent form asked the parents to sign "if you wish to have your child given the benefit of this new preventative."[11] It was also undetermined whether all the youngsters there would really inevitably contract hepatitis. It is possible that some parents were gently coerced into agreeing by being offered a place for their children in the research unit when places in the regular unit were not available. An explanation was needed that the United States Army Medical Research and Development Command was one of the funders of the study. Further, the type of protocol they provided was not discussed.

The most interesting question arises, however, if these more obvious questions were put to rest by making whatever adjustments necessary to assure that the parents were giving a consent of unassailable quality. A fundamental ethical problem would remain even if parents were given all the relevant information for consent to be informed and the consent were obtained in a completely non-coercive manner. Is it ethically defensible to experiment on human subjects who can benefit from the experiment only because of their miserable social condition? There are several alternative answers to this question.

One alternative is to ban all interventions for the purpose of gaining knowledge on subjects who cannot adequately give their consent. This would include children, some mental patients, and, under some views, the further categories of prisoners, armed forces personnel, low-income and ethnic populations with limited medical alternatives, and patients hospitalized for conditions not related to the experiment.

This view has serious problems. According to this view, for example, no research on children, infants, and individuals suffering from those types of mental disorders that by their very nature preclude full and informed consent could ever be justified. This would mean that such individuals would be unable to benefit from studies that investigate problems that are specific to these populations, since such studies would have to use these subjects in question. One way to test the reasonableness of this view is to ask how one would want such a group to be treated assuming that oneself will someday be unable to consent. It seems reasonable to conclude that a person imagining this hypothetical situation would not want all such research banned.

A second alternative takes the opposite view, namely, that the interests of the individual patient should be subordinated to the greater good of society. This view, if taken to its logical extreme, would not see any injustice in using a disadvantaged subject population to conduct a study even if *no* advantages or even disadvantages accrued to the subject. As long as the goal sought was thought to be significant enough, it seems this view would permit us to use others exclusively as a means to achieve our goal. This view cannot even consistently require us to always obtain consent since according to this method of justification, as long as the good to be obtained for society is important enough, there is no reason why in principle this consent requirement could not be waived. The flaws of this view are so apparent that a refutation is hardly needed. Cases such as this one make clear the serious problems raised by applying the principle of beneficence alone. If the only objective were to produce as much good as possible, then studies such as that at Willowbrook probably could be justified easily. In fact, if maximizing net benefit is the only objective, then the disadvantaged subject population could be used in the study even if *no* benefits of improved sanitation and health care accrued to them. As long as the goal sought was thought to be significant enough, this view would permit us to use others exclusively as a means.

A third alternative has emerged in the ethics of human-subjects research that offers more promise in solving our problem since it requires at least some consideration of the welfare of the subject as well as other potential beneficiaries. On March 8, 1983, Department of Health and Human Services issued regulations pertaining to the use of children as research subjects.[12] They divide research that involves more than minimal risk into three categories: research presenting the prospect of direct benefit to the individual subjects, research with no prospect of direct benefit to individual subjects, but likely to yield generalizable knowledge about the subject's disorder or condition, and research not otherwise approvable which presents an opportunity to understand, prevent, or alleviate a serious problem affecting the health or welfare of children. In each case limits are placed on the risks to which subjects incapable of consenting may be exposed. These limits make sense only if we focus on the unique ethical claims of the individual as well as the contributions of the research to society.

The Willowbrook study might conceivably be classified under any of the three categories. Even considering the controlled exposure to hepatitis alone, the research procedure might be considered of direct benefit to the subject. It is not clear whether the benefits of increased sanitation and better health care that are part of the research could count as "direct benefit to the individual subjects." If they do, then the case for the acceptability of the study is easy to make. Under such circumstances the risk must be justified by the anticipated benefit to the subject, which it surely is.

On the other hand, the research could be considered to offer no prospect of *direct* benefit to individual subjects. It could be argued that giving hepatitis cannot be considered a benefit at all and that the other ancillary benefits—the improved sanitation and living conditions—are indirect benefits. When there is no prospect of direct benefit, the research must involve no more than a "minor increase over minimal risk." In this case a great deal depends on how risks are determined. It would be possible to assess net risks to the subject, that is the net of the anticipated harm in comparison with the potential benefits including the indirect ones. If that approach were used, the Willowbrook investigator could claim, as he did, that the risks to the subjects were no more than a "minor increase over minimal." In fact, the benefits of the intervention reasonably far exceeded the anticipated harms. Again the research plausibly could be justified.

The third possibility is that the Willowbrook study could be classified as research not otherwise approvable that presents an opportunity to understand, prevent, or alleviate a serious problem affecting the health or welfare of children. In this case the research must be found by a panel of experts to offer a reasonable opportunity to further the understanding, prevention, or alleviation of a serious problem affecting the welfare of children and to make adequate provisions for assent of the children and permission of the parents or guardian. Surely the Willowbrook study could be designed to satisfy these criteria. It must also, however, be found to be conducted in accordance with sound ethical principles. Since it, in all likelihood, can be made to satisfy the principles of benefience, autonomy, and other ethical principles except justice, the real question is whether it is just.

It seems, therefore, that even if we focus specifically on the benefits and harms to the patient, the Willowbrook study could be justified according to the DHHS regulations regardless of the category in which the research were placed, if some preliminary adjustments were made to assure that adequately voluntary and informed parental permission was obtained and that the principle of justice is satisfied.

What is missed in all of this is the moral significance, if any, of the fact that the bulk of the benefits (whether we call them direct or indirect) are not inherently part of the research intervention and that no intervention would be necessary at all if proper conditions were provided in the first place. Does it make a moral difference whether the anticipated benefits are to result directly from the research procedure—as they would, for example, if a new antibiotic were to be tested on a child with an otherwise incurable infection—or, alternatively, they are given to subjects as a "compensation" or "accompaniment" for the risks undertaken. In the latter case the compensatory benefits could be offered independent of the research (although society does not appear to be prepared to make such an offer).

If these compensatory benefits not directly linked to the research intervention can be counted in the calculation of net benefit to the subject, then it would be possible to justify virtually any risk to the subject, provided the compensation were great enough. In fact, the worse off the subjects were, the easier it would be to justify using them in risky research. If researchers were fortunate enough to find and be able to use subjects on the verge of death by starvation who were without hope of any other social rescue, they would be justified in imposing any risk short of certain death provided they only supplied enough food for the subjects to live. The result of the intervention (including the compensatory benefits) would be a net benefit. Anything could be justified if the subject were miserable enough. Thus serious problems of justice seem to arise if one is permitted to take compensatory benefits into account since the people who will benefit the most and, therefore, be most easily justified as research subjects are those who are most miserable. Can we, as the DHHS regulations seem to imply, "take advantage" of the fact that certain potential subjects are miserable in order to justify recruiting them as subjects?

It is likely that there are important variables in answering that question that are not considered by the regulation writers. The first is whether other options are open to benefit the subjects who are in such a miserable situation. At the one extreme if a subject is miserable from an incurable disease, there is surely nothing wrong with offering a dangerous experimental intervention and counting even a small chance of success as a potential benefit. In such a situation there is no other possibility of benefitting the patient. We might even say that such an offer is "coercively attractive." Provided there is no other option available, making such an offer seems to violate neither autonomy nor justice.

By contrast if other safe, simple, and sure remedies were available to the one making the offer, such an offer would surely be ethically unacceptable. A researcher who had the only source of penicillin available, but refused to make it available to a patient suffering from a condition amenable to penicillin, would be acting unethically were he to offer the patient a choice between an experimental antibiotic and death. Offers to benefit people who are in a miserable situation are justified if there is no alternative available to benefit the persons so miserable. Whether they are also justified in cases where there exist alternative ways of relieving the misery is a more complicated question.

The interesting fact about the Willowbrook experiment is that there clearly are other alternatives available—cleaning up the problematic sanitary and health-care conditions. The problem is that such cleanup is not normally thought of as being a responsibility of the researcher qua researcher. Were the potential investigator the administrator of the unsanitary institution—or even better—the legislator who refused to vote for funds to improve sanitation at the institution, it seems clear there is a special professionally related obligation that would make taking advantage of the subjects' misery particularly offensive. On the other hand, if the subject were an average citizen with no related professional responsibilities, abandoning one's life plan in order to improve the conditions at the institution would be noble, but hardly one's strict moral duty. It would be supererogatory.

This consideration raises two intriguing problems in determining the ethics of experimentation such as the Willowbrook research. First, does merely being a trained physician with specific knowledge of the conditions at the institution generate a special duty to improve those conditions? For example, assuming the investigators are specialists in virology and not particularly specialized in the care of the retarded or any of the clinical professions relevant to the institution, to what extent do they have a duty to stop their research and devote their time to the cleanup? A case can be made that, simply by their professional competence and knowledge they have more of an obligation than other citizens, but it seems hardly reasonable to conclude they have a strict moral duty to abandon their research in order to help the Willowbrook residents. After all, investigators have already given their lives to helping a group of poorly off people, the sufferers from hepatitis. Perhaps by the mere fact that they are health professionals in New York with specific knowledge of Willowbrook's conditions they are bound to act to some extent, but it hardly seems reasonable that they must abandon all their work to give their lives to Willowbrook reform. As members of their profession with their knowledge the researchers cannot be diverted totally from their present project.

The second question is more problematical. It asks whether by proposing to take advantage of the misery of the residents, the researchers gain any further special responsibility over and above that of being knowledgeable health professionals. By intervening directly into that environment they may gain a special responsibility not existing otherwise.

I suggest that how one answers this question depends upon how one answers a fundamental question of ethics. There are two views about how one should respond to what appears to be inevitable though hypothetically preventable evil. One group, we might call them the realists, say that the ethically correct thing to do in a situation is to act according to the rules or judgments that will lead to the most right of the realistically possible outcomes, recognizing that the world is not perfect. Such persons acknowledge evil in the world and try to make the best of a bad situation. They support wars if (and only if) the wars are just; they maximize the welfare of the poor by permitting them to omit vitally needed health care if some other need is greater; they opt for what Ernst Troeltsch would call "relative natural law," the moral law that is most appropriate for a real world with its moral imperfections.[13]

Others, who we might call idealists, reject this approach. They say that the ethically correct thing to do is to act according to the rules or judgments that would lead to the most right outcome if other persons and institutions were doing what was morally correct. These are the people Troeltsch identifies as insisting on what he calls "absolute natural law." Insofar as their own behavior is concerned, they will strive to make it conform to the ideal even if they recognize others elsewhere in the system may make their behavior lead to a less than ideal outcome. These people may well be pacifists; they will probably insist on delivering a fair share of health care to the poor even if they cannot deal with broader questions of equitable distribution of resources.

I suspect that in the case of the Willowbrook research, if everything were done to make the proposed research as ethical as possible (by improving the quality of the parental permission, minimizing the risks to the subjects, etc.), there would still be a moral division between the realists and the idealists. The realists would say that the facts are that the Willowbrook children are at greater risk from the custodial wards than they are from the research even though the research purposely exposes them to hepatitis. The realists would insist that the researcher maximize the welfare of the children—by conducting the experiment.

The idealist, on the other hand, would say that insofar as the researchers are directly involved with the injustice of the treatment of those children, they cannot take advantage of it even if doing so would make the children better off in comparison with their alternative. In their own lives they should behave the way they would in an ethically just world, which is one in which these miseries of the children would not exist and therefore, one in which the research would not be possible.

Assuming that the researchers are not obligated to improve the Willowbrook situation simply by virtue of the fact that they are professionals with specific knowledge of the miserable situation, a case can be made that they at least have a duty not to take advantage of that misery to fulfill their agenda even if in doing so they could make the subjects better off. That case, however, is not obvious. Once one makes preliminary adjustments to assure that communication with parents is of high quality and that the children are exposed to only the minimal necessary risk, the realists will support those who take advantage of misery in order to improve the lot of the least well-off. In doing so they will have to be very sure that there is no realistic possibility of improvement in underlying conditions. The fact is that soon after the

Willowbrook experiments ended conditions improved dramatically through public outcry and political action. This suggests that researchers defending research on the grounds that it benefits others who are, given the realities of an imperfect world, inevitably in a miserable situation need to assess their facts very carefully. If they and the institutional review boards that must approve their research are convinced that subjects are otherwise inevitably doomed to misery, these realists would push forward and approve the research. Those who remain ethically uneasy at this point, those who resist approval even though it would relieve the apparently inevitable misery of a miserable group of subjects, must be making the moves of the ethical idealists. They must be insisting that it is unethical to take advantage of the fact that even though a problem could, in theory, be corrected, people in the real world are too callous, too insensitive, too unethical to do so. That, in the end, may not be an irrational stance to take.

The Problem of Preliminary Data: Longitudinal Studies, Sequential Design, and Grant Renewals

Another group of problems in the design and conduct of research that arise once one views the patient as a partner focuses more on the principle of autonomy rather than the principle of justice. One of these could be called the preliminary data problem.

Longitudinal studies, protocols involving sequential design, and grant renewals share one characteristic. They all involve generating and evaluating preliminary data before the research is successfully completed. They pose a serious problem for IRBs and anyone else interested in the ethics of human-subjects research. The data trickle in a bit at a time. It is good scientific procedure and essential to the protection of human subjects to examine those data as they appear to make sure that subjects are not being exposed to serious or unnecessary risks and that time and other resources are not being wasted.

Preliminary data also pose serious problems, however. Every time a new piece of information is generated the risks and benefits of a piece of research change slightly. In a controlled clinical trial, after every dose of the active compound or the placebo, the researcher knows or could know slightly more than before. The problem becomes most dramatic in the sophisticated techniques of sequential design.

The techniques of sequential experimentation are rooted in complex statistical concepts. They have their origins in the 1940s and developed into powerful pharmacological tools in the next two decades.[1] In sequential design the observations are examined as they become available. A decision is made to end the trial at the precise point where the accumulating results become significant.

There is a generally accepted moral imperative not to expose subjects unnecessarily to randomization or to a treatment that can be shown to be inferior. The techniques of sequential design have the attractive potential of signalling a significant result as soon as possible and therefore eliminating any unnecessary exposure of subjects to inferior treatments. Unfortunately, since the data are analyzed sequentially, the researcher also knows when a treatment course is very close to being shown to be inferior or superior at any predetermined level of significance. He or she may be shooting for a .05 significance level, but at some point be able to say that arm A of the study is superior to arm B at only a .06 level.

Although the technique is ethically imperative to avoid unnecessary exposure of subjects to inferior treatments, sooner or later an even more difficult ethical dilemma arises. Someone must ask if reasonable subjects would want to be told that treatment A is looking like it will prove superior, that at probability levels slightly below an acceptable significance level, the researcher could say that treatment A is superior based on presently available data. While such "almost significant" data are not satisfactory to the pharmacologist, they may be very interesting indeed to the patient whose life or welfare hangs on getting the most effective treatment course. Often the patient will not be able to wait until the definitive data are in.

The problem of preliminary data is not limited to protocols using formal techniques of sequential design. Although statistical techniques such as sequential design ought to be used whenever possible to minimize the risk to subjects, a similar moral problem of preliminary data arises whenever a longitudinal study is being conducted. It arises in an inescapable way whenever an IRB acts on a grant renewal for an ongoing research project. By year two of a study knowledge has often accrued from year one. Some IRBs are now routinely requiring a report on all such data at the time continuation approval is given for renewal of the project grant. At the very least the IRB needs to have such data to fulfill its responsibility to provide continual monitoring of the research to assure that human subjects have their rights and welfare protected. Thus, the first question of longitudinal studies is the obligation of the IRB to review new data as they are available.

But once the IRB has the data, it must face the question of whether subjects ought to be told the more recent findings. It is becoming increasingly clear that subjects of research, if they are to be treated as autonomous agents who are full partners in the research process, have a right to be told all information that the reasonable subject would find material in deciding to participate in the study. Moreover, it is well established that the alternative courses of action and their relative risks and benefits must be conveyed to the subject. It seems that knowledge that at the present time treatment A is producing better (but not yet statistically significantly better) results than treatment B is the kind of information that a subject might find very material to his or her decision to participate. The question has particularly practical implications in those cases where subjects have the option of declining to participate in the study. In these cases they may be able to obtain the potentially more effective treatment on the outside. If a semi-randomized design is adopted, as suggested in chapter 9, they may even be able to obtain it within the research context. It seems as if the IRB would reasonably have the duty to insist that the consent information be changed as new data become available. Only then could each patient assess the currently available data before deciding whether to consent to a randomization.

Several years ago a multicenter trial was underway to test the hypothesis that aspirin was more effective than placebos in preventing recurrent myocardial infarction.[2] As the early data came in, aspirin began to appear more effective. Those studies made clear that additional studies would be required to confirm or refute this conclusion. Nevertheless someone who at that point in history had suffered myocardial infarction and had been selected as a candidate for the multicenter study might, if properly informed, reasonably have decided to decline to participate in the study in order to begin taking aspirin on his or her own. In this case the collaboration of the physician would not even have been required, although medical supervision would certainly seem wise. In other cases the withdrawal from the study in order to choose an apparently preferable course of action would require the cooperation of medical professionals either in or outside of a protocol. Often, however, especially when the experimental group is beginning to appear no better or even worse than the routine therapy, physicians would be readily available to provide the routine treatment should the patient decide to decline to participate in the study.

The decision to choose one of the treatment arms rather than randomization will depend on many factors including the individual idiosyncrasies of specific potential subjects. Some patients may want to take every possible opportunity to combat the cancer with the latest chemotherapy regimen even if it appears only marginally more successful and produces significant toxicity. Another patient might decline the randomization into the protocol in order to opt for the more conservative conventional treatment. The decision would also depend upon the latest available information about the relative benefits and harms of the experimental and conventional regimens. Subjects would reasonably want to know the latest available data.

They should, of course, realize that data that are only approaching statistical significance can be misleading. But opting for the conventional therapy would be far more plausible if the null hypothesis were approaching an adequate level of statistical significance. It seems impossible to escape the conclusion that reasonable subjects would often want to know the latest available data generated by the early phases of the study. In sequential designs they would often want to know the current degree of certainty with which the researcher could say that there is no reason to prefer one course of action over the other. In any longitudinal study, whether it uses strict sequential analysis or not, subjects might reasonably want to know what the data are beginning to look like. At least those entering year two of a study are in a very different position from those entering year one. In fact, if, after several years of a longitudinal study, no change is made in the consent form and no new information is transmitted to the potential subject, the IRB is justified in asking why. If no information of interest has come from earlier subjects, then it is unclear what could justify a continuation of the study. Even if such a continuation could be justified, the fact that we cannot tell whether the new procedure is any better than the old one would certainly be a piece of information of interest to patients. At the very least, in every longitudinal study the IRB must from time to time review preliminary data and assess the new benefit/harm ratios.

THE IMPACT OF SCIENTIFIC VALIDITY

All of this suggests that each subject or at least various groups of subjects ought to get information slightly different—slightly updated—from the previous subject. At least year-two subjects ought to get different information from year-one subjects. But quite obviously this wreaks havoc for scientific validity. The most obvious problem is that often virtually no reasonable patient/subject would volunteer to be randomized if he or she were told that the researchers are approaching the point where they can conclude that one treatment is better than the other. In fact consenting to be randomized in such situations when serious issues are at stake could be *prima facie* evidence that the patient is not consenting freely or not consenting in an informed state. It appears that researchers would perpetually be doomed to getting almost significant findings and then reasonable subjects would decline to participate. No significant conclusions could ever be reached.

The problem is more subtle. In the early stages of such studies only minor trends will have emerged so that subjects might reasonably consent to be randomized even if they were told that the early results were beginning to show one course slightly better than the other. But if each subject is told of the latest findings, the scientific goal of minimizing the difference between the two groups will be jeopardized. Certainly subjects should enter the study with similar expectations and similar prior knowledge of what side effects are anticipated. If, however, after several trials an unanticipated side effect emerges and consent procedures are modified to convey the newly found side effects to future subjects, the new subjects will not be strictly comparable.

What is ideal ethically is a disaster scientifically. Following ethical principles would result in no two subjects being comparable and many studies could not be carried to the point where statistically significant results are produced. This is the essential problem the IRB must face.

Four possible solutions come to mind. First, an IRB might convince itself that reasonable subjects might not really want to know the preliminary findings. They could conclude that data that are not statistically significant would not be interesting to the subject. In fact, the IRB could go even further and argue that if one treatment arm has not been shown to be statistically significantly better than another there really is nothing to communicate. An IRB member might argue that he or she really does not know that aspirin prevents repeated myocardial infarction, that it would be irresponsible to transmit information upon which a patient started a course of treatment based on preliminary, possibly erroneous suggestions.

It certainly would have been irresponsible of an IRB to require a researcher to imply to a subject that in 1974 after the intial study aspirin was known to decrease myocardial infarction risk when no such significant evidence was available. It would be wrong to publish a scientific paper to that effect or to conclude that such a superiority has been proved. But subjects are interested in a very different kind of significance than the scientist. While a .06 significance level may count for almost nothing in a scientific paper, it would be very interesting to a subject. Some subjects would find some preliminary trends in data very significant—not significant in the statistical sense, but significant in the more traditional sense of being important, important enough so that one could rationally choose a course of action that would maximize the chance of a good medical outcome. Personal significance of the data for patients could be quite different from its scientific significance for the researcher. IRB members would be fooling themselves if they concluded that all data that are not statistically significant are of no interest to subjects.

The justification of nondisclosure would have to be that the reasonable subject would not want the information. When this is truly the case, this justification might provide a way out of the dilemma of the IRB having to reevaluate and rewrite the consent after each subject. Perhaps the reasonable person would not care in some cases to have every last piece of new data, provided they were not going to have any real impact on his or her decision. Limiting IRB review to periodic examination of the new data and limiting consent-form revisions to those periods would be justified but only in those cases in which a reasonable subject would not want the new data as they become available. A reasonable subject on the other hand might want the data from the latest subject if those data were dramatic, if they would reasonably have some impact on his or her decision to participate in the study.

A second possible course would be to admit as done above, that such preliminary findings would be interesting to some subjects and that they might even rationally influence their decision to participate in the study. Yet, an IRB might conclude, nevertheless, that the value of the research is so great and the necessity of achieving scientifically valid and statistically significant results so important that the potential benefits to society outweigh the violation of the subject's right to the information necessary for an informed consent, i.e., the information a subject would find material in deciding whether to participate in the study.

This argument from social benefit for withholding the preliminary findings that accumulate in the early phases of studies provides a logically coherent justification for the common practice of not changing the consent form and the information transmitted during a longitudinal study or a sequentially designed experiment. An IRB that withheld the information on those grounds would at least be consistent.

Once one realizes, however, that this is information that many reasonable subjects would want in deciding whether to participate and that in some of these cases the choice is literally a matter of life and death, the IRB does not seem to be justified in its defense of using social usefulness as a definitive justification for compromising the subject's right to consent. Since Nuremberg, Western society has accepted that benefits to society are a necessary condition for justifying research on human subjects. At Nuremberg we abandoned the traditional position of medical professionals, namely that benefit to the patient alone justifies exposing the patient to risks, but Nuremberg also made it dramatically clear that it was not benefits to society alone that was the decisive criterion either. Other conditions must also be satisfied, in particular the requirement of adequate consent grounded in the principle of autonomy. Thus, to offset what would otherwise be an intolerable violation of the integrity and autonomy of the patient or subject, Nuremberg and all significant commentators on human experimentation since that time have insisted on the principle of consent. Requiring consent ensures that the subject is treated as an end in himself, i.e., as a being capable of self-determination, rather than as merely a means to a researcher's end.

These considerations justify American law and the DHHS regulations that forbid withholding crucial information from a subject that he or she would be likely to find material in deciding whether to participate in a study.

DHHS regulation imposes seven requirements on IRBs in their review of research where human subjects are at risk.[3] They must establish that the risks to the subject are minimized and reasonable in relation to anticipated benefits to the subject and the importance of the knowledge that may reasonably be expected to result. (Social benefits are indeed a legitimate concern.) But they must also assure that subject gives an adequately informed consent. Social usefulness alone cannot justify withholding the preliminary data even if withholding it would provide the crucial subjects necessary to establish statistically that an intervention is more effective than its alternatives. That is at least the state of the law. Most would conclude it is the state of our ethics as well.

The third option the IRB has is to insist that the subject be given the preliminary data. This might be done in full awareness that doing so will compromise scientific ideals. But depending on the specifics of the research, great harm may really not be done to the validity of the study. Subjects may not strictly be comparable in as pure a way as they would have been if the preliminary information were withheld from later subjects in a longitudinal study. But often the conclusions reached will be sufficiently clear that no reasonable person would question whether the newer information to the later subjects changed the results in any significant way. A perfect scientific methodology is not always the decisive criterion. An IRB will normally incorporate members within its composition that value other goods as well as perfect scientific methodology. It is probably healthy if at least some IRB members in a body committed to protecting the subject incorporate other values in their decision-making besides scientific values.

Sometimes, however, the new information will make a successful completion of the study impossible. The final subjects to give the sequentially designed experiment significance will not be obtainable. The newly discovered side effects will so change the character of the subject's participation that he or she is in reality not comparable to the earlier subjects.

There is a fourth option that occurs that takes into consideration these special cases. I think they will arise much less often than at first it would appear. But if the IRB is convinced that such is or will be the case in a protocol before it, it might consider permitting researchers to ask subjects to consent to have certain key pieces of information withheld.

This solution is rather like that proposed for protocols necessarily involving deception. In this case, however, the key information being withheld can usually be disclosed to the subject without making the research logically impossible to complete. In this way it is like informing a subject that he is being randomized, that is, that he or she will not be told one key piece of information—the treatment he or she will be receiving. Informing a subject that there will be randomization without telling him or her which group he or she is entering, is certainly withholding a piece of information that the subject might find meaningful. It certainly is a compromise with the principle of consent. It is really a consent to less than full disclosure. As such most would find the selective withholding acceptable, morally and legally. Likewise, some cases of consent to have the latest data withheld might be morally acceptable.

This is not to say, however, that data can always justifiably be withheld. Perhaps it could not even be withheld with the consent of the subject. The IRB will have to monitor withheld preliminary data carefully. Such subjects would be placing a special trust in the IRB and the researcher. In some cases the newly developed preliminary information may simply have to be transmitted to the subjects. This may have to be done even before the study has reached a level of significance that would satisfy researchers. Newly discovered, but not yet statistically significant, differences in mortality between treatment groups may not warrant waiting until a high level of significance is reached. The disclosure of the preliminary data unearthed in the longitudinal study or sequential design may have to be disclosed to new subjects even if it jeopardizes the study itself. The task of the IRB is to assure that the rights of these new subjects are protected as well as assuring that the risks to them are justified by the potential benefits to the subject and society.

The problem of preliminary data is an intriguing one, one that IRBs and scholars working on the ethics of human experimentation have been troubled by for some time. It is perplexing that the techniques of longitudinal study and sequential design that were developed out of a moral imperative to protect subjects from undue risk have in turn left us with a new moral dilemma.

These four strategies for coping with the preliminary data problem are successful in varying degrees and in varying circumstances. If I am correct in insisting that the principle of beneficence—of maximizing aggregate benefit—can never override autonomy, then it is never acceptable on grounds of scientific need to withhold preliminary data that persons would reasonably want. In some cases it may be reasonable to conclude that subjects would really not want the preliminary data. Such a determination would be difficult; it may require empirical evidence such as that suggested in the next chapter. If, however, it can plausibly be argued that subjects would not want the data, then such data could justifiably be withheld. In a number of cases the strategy of getting subjects to consent to having these data withheld may be the most plausible course. Provided the data are not of crucial importance to a rational decision, subjects could, if they see themselves as an integral part of the scientific enterprise, sacrifice their desire to know for the good of the science. In some cases where the information really is crucial such consent to ignorance will be morally unacceptable. In those cases the research will have to be modified to take the requirements of adequately informed consent, including information about preliminary data, into account.

CHAPTER TWELVE

Informed Consent: The Use of Lay Surrogates to Determine How Much Information Should Be Transmitted

Richard Winer, Robert M. Veatch, Victor W. Sidel, and Morton Spivack

Increasing ethical and legal complexity in the requirements that patients and subjects of research give an adequately informed consent has made it more and more difficult for physicians, researchers, and institutional review boards to determine precisely what must be disclosed to subjects for a consent to be reasonable and adequate. It is becoming increasingly clear that personal estimates by clinicians and researchers about what information ought to be transmitted will give widely varying and sometimes inappropriate answers. There is a need for more sophisticated methods of determining what information should be transmitted to patients and subjects and how much of that information is retained.

Clinicians, researchers, and the institutional review boards in hospitals and research centers make judgments on clinical care and research projects as well as on the informed consent related to those activities. The members of institutional review boards, for instance, make decisions for subjects of research about how much a reasonable person should be told about the nature and purpose of the experiments. Yet, those decisions are not always acceptable to each and every subject because certain data are more important to one person than the next. Problems arise because professional people sitting on the boards may not be able to assess correctly the laymen's views. Ultimately, though, subjects are asked to sign forms authorizing their participation in the study. Through this entire process the subjects have had little, if any, input to the committees concerning their own personal beliefs about what they would like to be told. This points out the need for additional empirical data on what information may be considered appropriate to obtain an adequately informed consent.

One area that needs to be examined in this regard is the impact of consent and the recall ability of the subjects. A few attempts have been made to ascertain patient or subject responses to informed consent. Alfidi's first two studies involved patients undergoing angiography.[1,2] After reading a consent form that detailed risks of the procedure, the patients were asked if they appreciated receiving information about those risks. They were also queried about any change of mind about the procedure after being presented with the risks. The patients were additionally asked if others should receive the same information. Almost eighty-five percent of the patients appreciated receiving the information. Approximately seventy-five percent of the patients felt that all patients should receive the information; yet twenty-seven percent of the patients were made less comfortable by the information. Only ten out of eight hundred patients in the studies refused to consent to the angiography. The third study included a segment of the consent form asking the patients if they wanted information concerning risks and complications of the study.[3] Only about one-third of the patients stated that they wished to be apprised of the risks. The question itself was so general that it poses other questions, such as the determination of which risks should be divulged and what should be done about the differences in opinion concerning the disclosure.

A study by Robinson and Merav involved taping of the preoperative interview and subsequent questioning of cardiac patients four to six months after open heart survey.[4] The tape was replayed, and the items discussed in the original interview were charted for quick accessibility before the reinterview. The survey revealed that the patients averaged a general recall of twenty-nine percent of the information presented in the informed-consent interview. After some suggestion of correct answers and a "point-by-point" review of the items in the original interviews, the patients were still able to recall an average of forty-two percent of the details. The topics discussed were the diagnosis and nature of the illness, the proposed operation, the risks of the operation, potential complications, benefits of the procedure, and alternative procedures. Reporting findings in terms of percent recall without analysis of the specific nature of the questions asked makes interpretation of the findings difficult.

Another area of discussion dealing with consent upon which more data are needed is the problem of what information should be provided for a consent to be adequately informed. Until 1969, courts generally held that information that should be disclosed was limited to those disclosures which a reasonable medical practitioner would make under like circumstances.[5] However, the tide has turned in some jurisdictions in recent years. Deciding what a reasonable person would want to know has transcended using the medical profession as the reference standard. Now many courts have recognized that the critical question is what the reasonable layperson would want to know for his or her consent to be adequately informed. This means that even though there exists a consensus among professionals in the field that a particular risk should not be disclosed, it is still an open question whether the reasonable layperson would want to know about that risk. This "reasonable person" concept has been used in many legal determinations. The California court in *Berkey* v. *Anderson* in 1969 recognized potential differences between professional and lay views and declared: "We cannot agree that the matter of informed consent must be determined on the basis of medical testimony any more than that expert testimony of the practice is determinative in any other case involving a fiduciary relationship. We agree with appellant that a physician's duty to disclose is not governed by the standard practice of the physician's community, but it is a duty imposed by law which governs his conduct in the same manner as others in a similar fiduciary relationship. To hold otherwise would permit the medical profession to determine its own responsibilities. . . ."[6]

Since then legal opinions have almost unanimously pointed to the conclusion that even if professionals agree that the information is not required for an adequately informed consent, the reasonable person—as measured by the opinion of a jury—can still decide that it is required. In *Cobbs* v. *Grant,* the court decided that a "mini-course in medical science" is not essential, but nevertheless concluded that a patient should be adequately told of risks that could markedly affect his decision to consent to the procedure. The amount of information given to the patient "must be measured by the patient's need, and that need is whatever information is material to the decision."[7]

The court in *Wilkinson* v. *Vesey* followed the Cobbs track on materiality. Recognizing that a reasonable disclosure varies from instant to instant, the court stated, "Materiality may be said to be the significance a reasonable person, in what the physician knows or should know is his patient's position, would attach to the disclosed risk or risks in deciding whether to submit or not to submit to surgery or treatment."[8]

Likewise, in *Canterbury* v. *Spence,*[9] the judge reported that "the test for determining whether a particular peril must be divulged is its materiality to the patient's decision: all risks potentially affecting the decision must be unmasked." The judge also pointed out that the physician must present information regardless of what the standard in the medical community might be at the moment. "Respect for the patient's right of self-determination on particular therapy demands a standard set by law rather than one which physicians may or may not impose upon themselves." Self-determination or autonomy is one principle underlying the requirement that informed consent be obtained. In attempting to decide how much information needs to be divulged, one must consider what information a patient will need in exercising self-determination. At times the level and type of information that must be disclosed under the standard of promoting self-determination may be different from the amount of information that would have to be disclosed if the standard were the protection of the patient from harm or the protection of society's interests.[10] It may also be different from the level of information that would have to be disclosed if the standard were the current practice of medical professionals in the community.

In the area of consent for protection of subjects of research, in an effort to evaluate questions of consent by the standard of what the reasonable person would want to know, institutional review boards have gradually added laypeople and interdisciplinary professionals to their memberships. The attempt to include such people might be helpful, but it cannot provide a definite answer to the question of what information should be presented to a subject. The laypeople on the board are usually specialists in some area, so they are not really true representatives of the lay community. Some lay members may, in fact, have more rigorous standards of what information must be transmitted than the subjects would have. Also, when decisions are made by committees involving both research professionals and laypeople, the net result, to the extent the two groups have identifiable positions, is likely to be a compromise between the two groups' viewpoints. Only by accident will that compromise replicate the views held by reasonable future research subjects.[11]

Proposals have been made to bring the layperson into a more active role in determining what the reasonable person wants to know. One such method is the surrogate system of consent examined by Fost.[12] He explained that "the essence of this process is to obtain a response from individuals who in fact are not candidates for investigative or therapeutic procedures, but who are asked to behave as if they were." Fost attempted to measure responses from people who could be presented the more pertinent facts of the procedure and could give more candid and diverse responses than those who might actually need to make such a decision. A possible study involving umbilical artery catheterization in very ill premature infants was presented for their approval to sixteen parents of children not needing such potential treatment. Eight of the sixteen parents leaned toward consent for the mock study. Four leaned toward refusal and four subjects decided not to participate in this hypothetical procedure.

The surrogate-recipient-panel concept was also discussed by the National Immunization Work Group on Consent[13] in a section dealing with what should be disclosed in immunization programs. A reasonable-person standard could possibly be better implemented through sampling of and discussion with surrogate participants. The panel's work would be beneficial in obtaining *ipso facto* lay judgments of what should or should not be disclosed to future subjects. In this way, a case may be presented to a jury-like body that can render its decision before anyone is involved in the study.

To test the feasibility of using lay surrogates to determine what subjects should be told about research interventions, these issues were explored as part of a larger interview survey of volunteer blood donors. Institutional review boards are from time to time asked to approve protocols where blood obtained from the institution's blood bank will be used for research. The question arises: How much should donors be told about the possibility that their blood will be used for research? This is an example of the general problem of determining how much research subjects should be told. We decided to investigate whether blood donors would allow some or all of their donation to be used for research, to determine if the blood donors would want to provide informed consent for research use, to find out if the blood donors would want to know about the research in order to have sufficient information to supply such consent, to determine a preferred method of obtaining consent for the use of blood for research, to determine how sex, age, education, or social class affects these wishes on the part of the donor, and to relate these findings to the principle of self-determination and the concept of the lay surrogate panel.

METHODS

Two hundred volunteer blood donors between the ages of seventeen and sixty-four at the blood bank of a large teaching hospital in New York City were asked to permit an interview during the "rest period" following their donation. All donors had signed a hospital blood bank "consent card" before the donation, and those donors belonging to a blood program also filled out and signed a Greater New York Blood Program consent form. The hospital card stated, "I hereby grant permission to . . . to draw approximately one pint of blood from me, to be used in such manner as the hospital may deem desirable." Some donors had been asked and had consented to allowing a small amount (25ml) of additional blood to be taken for research; these donors signed another form authorizing the supplemental blood drawing.

The research protocol and the informed-consent procedure for the study had been approved by the hospital's institutional review board. The subjects were told that the questions concerned their feelings about giving blood, using the blood for research rather than for transfusion, and consenting to such procedures. The donors were asked to select their answer to each question from a list of possible answered typed on a card. Some questions required "yes" or "no" answers. The range of answers for other questions varied from "definitely yes" to "definitely not" or from "very necessary" to "very unnecessary." The donors were also invited to ask any questions at any time during the interview. All interviews were conducted by the same person. The last fifty donors were asked additional questions about the sufficiency of the hospital consent card as a consent for research use of part or all of the blood.

RESULTS

Of the 200 donors interviewed, 198 remembered signing the consent card and 92 percent of those recalling signing felt that signing the card was either "necessary" or "very necessary" (Table 1). Twenty-nine percent of the donors, however, failed to recall that the card said the pint of blood could be "used in such manner as the hospital may deem desirable." They could not recall this statement even though they were asked specifically if they remembered that piece of information and the question usually came only thirty minutes after the card itself was signed.

When the donors were presented with a hypothetical situation involving their permission for use of some or all of the blood for research, they were told to suppose that enough blood was available for transfusion purposes. Thus people could answer the questions strictly on the basis of allowing their blood to be used for research rather than being forced to make a choice between research and depriving patients of needed blood. Under these conditions, 95 percent of the donors stated they would "definitely" or "probably" not mind if a small amount—no more than two teaspoonsful—of blood would be used by a medical scientist in an experiment which might help patient care (Table 2). A lesser percent of donors, 81%, felt the same way about the use of all of the blood for such purposes (Table 3). Although these percentages are large, they indicate that there is a certain amount of objection to use of blood for research even if there were adequate blood available for therapeutic purposes. This is true even though the donors had signed a card saying they would permit their blood to be "used in such manner as the hospital may deem desirable."

The last fifty donors interviewed were included in a group that was asked if the existing consent card statement that the hospital could use the blood as it deemed "desirable" was sufficient for them to consent to the use of their blood for research. In fact, the hospital did not use this general statement as consent for research; a separate detailed consent form was used if part or all the blood drawn was to be used in research. Thirteen of the fifty donors did not remember the statement on the card and were therefore not asked about the card's sufficiency. Of the thirty-seven donors who did answer the question, 70 percent believed the present card was sufficient if a very small amount of blood was used for research while 27 percent were not satisfied with the present statement (Table 4). Thus even though 95 percent of the total sample had no objection to the use of a small amount of their blood for research, among those who were further asked whether the present vague statement constituted an adequate consent, only 70 percent were satisfied. When asked if the present statement was adequate if all of the blood were to be used for research, the donors gave a similar response (Table 5). Although the proportions of general affirmative and negative answers were very close, there was a swing from "definitely yes" to "probably yes" responses and a swing from "probably not" to "definitely not" replies when the question was changed from a situation involving a small amount of the donation to all of the donation.

All 200 of the donors were asked whether a more specific statement referring to the possible use of blood in research or personal contact by the researcher to obtain consent would be more adequate. The personal contact was preferred by 26 percent if a small quantity of blood would be used and was preferred by 29 percent if all the blood was to be utilized in such a manner (Tables 6 and 7).

Of the 50 donors asked about the adequacy of the consent card, the 37 who remembered the statement were asked to express their preference among the current general statement, a more specific statement about research, and personal contact by the researcher as the best consent for blood use in research. The present statement was considered the best by about 50 percent if some of the blood were used for research; about 40 percent of all the donors liked the specific statement on research and the remaining 10 percent wanted the personal contact (Table 8). Even if all of the blood were to be used for research, the percentages remained about the same among those remembering the general statement (Table 9).

If a statement concerning research were on the card, 95 percent of the donors would still be as likely to donate if some of the blood would be used for research (Table 10), while 80 percent of the donors would be as likely to donate all of the blood for research (Table 11).

One of the reasons why consent to a specific research project might be favored over the use of a general authorization that the blood may be used for any purpose the hospital deems desirable is that some donors may have views about the purpose of the research. One of the elements specified by the Department of Health and Human Services as necessary for an informed consent is an explanation of the purpose of the research.[14] Any blanket consent for use of the blood for "purposes deemed desirable" would not comply with this requirement. A researcher, for instance, might propose a study of donated blood with a controversial objective such as an attempt to determine blood markers for anti-social behavior, to develop a blood test in pregnant women that could lead to late-term abortions, or to examine racial correlates of blood composition. A donor might object to the specific purpose of the study even though he might have no general objection to the use of his blood for research purposes.

There was a split of 52 to 47 percent in favor of being told for what research the blood would be used (Table 12). Those receiving the current general statement on the card of course would not be told such information. Nearly one-half of both the yes and no answers were "probably" answers reflecting a curiosity on the part of the donors, but not a definite feeling about being told or not being told about the research.

Specific sub-groups had significantly different opinions about research. The donors who gave blood to replenish blood used by particular patients showed more hesitancy about research than the donors who gave blood while members of a donation program even though their blood would not be used specifically for those particular patients. Although the two groups were basically not averse to research, a smaller percentage of donors for patients definitely were as likely to donate if some or all of their blood were to be used for research (29 and 19 percent, respectively). Similarly, first-time donors were less willing to donate if any of the blood went for research purposes. More first-time donors, however, were giving blood for specific patients. The patient donors also wanted to know for what research the blood would be used more than the donors for programs (61 to 43 percent).

A striking paradox occurred in the separate analysis of male and female donors. Men did not mind if blood would be used for research as much as the women. But almost 30 percent of the males liked the personal contact by the researcher if the blood would be used for research. One-seventh of the women wanted the personal discussion if some blood was to be used for research and 20 percent felt that way if all of the blood were to be used for research.

The youngest group of donors were most skeptical about the use of all of the donation for research. Only 44 percent in the 17–34-year-old age category definitely did not mind if all the blood would be used for research while no other age group was below 60 percent. Sixty-four percent of the 17–24-year-olds would be as likely to donate under those circumstances; more than 77 percent of each of the other groups felt the same way. Substantially more in the 17–24 category, 48 percent, felt the personal contact with the researcher was better than the specific statement about research on the consent card. Also, the younger the donors, the more they wanted to know for what research the blood would be used.

Some individuals gave interesting comments about the hospital's use of blood for research. One fireman represented many donors when he stated, "I don't want to be in a position to make that decision." Another firefighter followed, "If they need it, they need it." Several program members said that as long as their families were covered, they did not care what was done with the blood. One gentleman said, "I don't care what they [the hospital] do with it [the blood] as long as they don't paint the walls with it."

The type of consent used in such procedures was also mentioned by several donors. Some said the hospital could do what it wanted with the blood and the present statement was satisfactory. "If they feel it should go to research, it should go to research," commented a high-school teacher. But those desiring the specific statement about research were also emphatic. An accountant stated, "Research is cold, so they should mention that the blood might be used for research or patient care." Others believed that a statement about research should be "quite visible, either in bold type or pointed out by someone."

Some donors did not mind the use of blood for research if they were consulted by the researcher or, perhaps, by an agent of the researcher: "An individual has a chance to query as to the particulars." A person giving blood as part of a program said, "The verbal contact carries more weight and convinces the donor." A physician stated, "The contact gives more information and brings research out of the lab." A somewhat skeptical nineteen-year-old added, "The contact would be best because you could get more information out of them." Some of those interviewed thought the personal contact would be a nice idea, but that it was too unwieldy and difficult for a researcher to speak to every person who gave blood that was to be used for an experiment.

Institutional review boards are faced with determining what subjects should be told. This study was an investigation of a possible empirical method to determine what information subjects might want to know. A basic objective of such work is to minimize, if not eliminate, inadequately informed consents and develop methods of determining what patients and subjects find meaningful and necessary to know rather than what clinicians, researchers, and lay committee members think they would want to know or should know. A further problem is raised by the findings. Donors, patients, and subjects, like professionals, have differing views about what information they would find necessary or desirable for a consent to be adequately informed. While 56 percent of the donors said they would want to be told in advance of any discomforts that could arise during the course of a routine blood donation, 39 percent probably or definitely would not want to be told those discomforts. In responding to the question of what kind of consent would be adequate if blood were used for research purposes, 51 percent were satisfied with the general statement on the card if a very small amount of blood were to be used and 49 percent would have been satisfied if all the blood were to be used for research.

COMMENTS

The question arises what standard should be used for determining when reasonable people would want to know a piece of information? A major problem thus faces institutional review boards when presented with such data because there is not an extremely clear-cut response. If one hundred percent of the donors insisted on disclosure, there would be very little question about whether to disclose. Also, if only one percent favored the disclosure, there would be little hesitation in excluding the information under consideration. Trying to establish a percentage of potential subjects who want to be told something as a standard for determining that item's inclusion as part of the consent process is far from an easy task. Suggestions have ranged from five percent to a "majority rule" concept. It is not at all clear that this is a matter to be settled by majority rule. Some elements of information might be decided on an individual basis. After some risks were disclosed, subjects might be told, "There are some additional risks that we believe are less serious than the ones you have been told about. Would you like to hear some more?" This is adequate, however, only for oral, individually negotiated consents. There are serious problems of monitoring oral consents as well as pragmatic problems of providing the personnel to adjudicate each case of deciding what amount of information is adequate.

The ethical issue at stake is whether providing an excess of information is morally the equivalent of providing less information than necessary. We are convinced they are not morally equivalent. A person who does not receive information that would be material to his decision to participate in a therapeutic or research procedure is participating without informed consent. He is being deprived of his right to self-determination, a fundamental right long recognized as the basis of the consent requirement. On the other hand, providing more information than is necessary to make an informed judgment is a complicated matter. It may simply be an inconvenience to the subject and the professional. If the subject is excessively burdened by too much information, he may give instructions that he has received enough. If the procedure involves research intervention without direct therapeutic benefit, he may choose to withdraw from the research. Only when excessive information is so great that it actually limits the capacity of the individual to exercise self-determination would too much information be morally the equivalent of too little information in terms of the violation of the individual's right of self-determination. There may also be a legal problem in providing "too much" information in the therapeutic situation: If the patient is deterred from a potentially life-saving procedure and then dies, do his survivors have a case for a claim of "wrongful death"?

The moral problem paramount to this report is in the disclosure of information. Either some people will not be told information they would have wanted to know, or some people will have information forced upon them that they did not really desire. The utilitarian might state that the consent most sufficient for the most people should be used. But this could conceivably lead to one less than the majority of people having their wishes totally ignored. If receiving more information than necessary is morally preferable to being underinformed, leaning toward giving a little too much information is a better policy. (It also seems to be a prudent way to avoid legal liability for proceeding without adequate consent, although legal questions are not our present focus.) Yet, if a person specifically asks not to be told information, then the researcher should not have to divulge these facts.

Should the institutional review boards continue to try to make such decisions about what should be disclosed or should the lay community, including panels of surrogate subjects, play a larger role? We have found that a group of surrogate subjects can provide useful empirical data to researchers and research committees about what donors would like to be told. In the case of using blood from a blood bank for research, there is virtually no extra risk in using some blood or taking a small additional amount. But there are those who would prefer to give consent for such procedures and be told about the purposes of the research, as evidenced by results of the survey. Having someone discuss these purposes with the donor might be feasible just before the actual donation; however, getting in touch with a donor once he or she has left the blood bank might be very difficult. If the researcher would want to talk to the donor some time after the donation, he would have to look up information from the subject's records or consent card. There could be some accusation of an invasion of privacy or a breach of confidentiality.

One criticism of the surrogate-panel method of determining what information should be transmitted is that it could force upon actual subjects the consensus views of such a panel, assuming that such a consensus could be established. Some individual subjects may well differ from this consensus, wanting either more or less information than this consensus of reasonable people would call for. It seems to us that the burden shifts at this point. If individual, actual patients want more or less information based on their own needs, they have the responsibility of making this known to the researchers. Room should always be left for questioning. This precludes the notion that the decision-making process will be completely taken away from the actual subject. In the specific case we have studied, it would seem reasonable that a more specific statement about research be included on a consent card and that it be made known that a member of the research team is available to answer questions. A physician who personally speaks to his patient before an operation is supposedly providing a desirable and advantageous function. A consultation between subject and researchers might be equally beneficial.

This may create problems for researchers who want to use standard consent procedures. It might create problems in the example of consent for research use of donated blood for researchers who want to use particular kinds of blood stored in the blood bank and are not able for some reason to obtain the specific, negotiated consent of the donor prior to the donation. It might be possible to have a statement on the consent form that blood may be used for research purposes if, in the judgment of the institutional review board, it does not jeopardize patient care and the board can conceive of no reasonable objections to the use of the blood for research purposes. This would permit review of protocols where the purpose of the research might be objectionable to some donors.

Institutional review boards already discuss protocols on several levels, including risk/benefit relations and the informed consent. A surrogate-subject panel can lighten the load somewhat in the consent area by suggesting what information should be divulged and how it should be presented. At least two types of surrogate panels might be useful. First, as was demonstrated in this study, individuals drawn from the same pool as those who are potential subjects for a future study may answer questions about what percentage of people would find information necessary or desirable. For other questions, however, a more active surrogate panel might also be helpful. This panel could be made up of present and past hospital patients who could respond to more specific questions of physicians, researchers, and boards. If, for instance, the board wanted to know whether the total number of risks being considered for inclusion in a consent form was in aggregate so many that the subject would be more confused than enlightened, the present kind of survey would not be helpful, but a consulting panel on call might be very useful. There is room for a surrogate panel to act as a consultant to the review board. The surrogates are in a better position to determine what a reasonable person would want to know about a particular procedure or piece of research. From legal, technical, and ethical standpoints, questioning of surrogate patients and subjects may often be the most useful and most reliable method of answering difficult questions about informed consent.

TABLE 1

Which phrase best describes your feelings about having had to sign the consent card for a blood donation?

Response	Number	Percent
Very necessary	113	57.1
Necessary	69	34.8
Unimportant	9	4.5
Unnecessary	5	2.5
Very unnecessary	2	1.0
	198	99.9

(Did not remember signing the consent card—2)

TABLE 2

Would you mind if a very small amount (not more than two teaspoonfuls) of the blood you donated would be used for research purposes rather than for transfusion?

Response	Number	Percent
Definitely yes	2	1.0
Probably yes	4	2.0
Don't know	3	1.5
Probably not	36	18.0
Definitely not	155	77.5
	200	100.0

TABLE 3

Would you mind if all of the blood you donated would be used
for such research purposes rather than for transfusion?

Response	Number	Percent
Definitely yes	12	6.0
Probably yes	12	6.0
Don't know	13	6.5
Probably not	39	19.5
Definitely not	124	62.0
	200	100.0

TABLE 4

If a very small amount of the blood you donated would be
used for research, would the present card be sufficient
for you to give your consent?

Response	Number	Percent
Definitely yes	23	62.2
Probably yes	3	8.1
Don't know	1	0.7
Probably not	5	13.5
Definitely not	5	13.5
	37	98.0

(Did not remember statement on card about research—13)

TABLE 5

If all of the blood you donated would be used for research,
would the present card be sufficient for you to give
your consent?

Response	Number	Percent
Definitely yes	19	51.4
Probably yes	8	21.6
Don't know	0	0.0
Probably not	2	5.4
Definitely not	8	21.6
	37	100.0

(Did not remember statement on card about research—13)

TABLE 6

Which of the following two methods of obtaining consent do you consider more adequate? (IF NO TO QUESTION IN TABLE 2)

Response	Number	Percent
Statement on consent card that a very small amount of blood might be used for research rather than transfusion	142	73.2
Contact by the researcher for specific permission to use a very small amount of the blood for research	50	25.8
Don't know	2	1.0
	194	100.0

TABLE 7

Which of the following two methods of obtaining consent do you consider more adequate? (IF NO TO QUESTION IN TABLE 3)

Response	Number	Percent
Statement on consent card that all of the blood might be used for research rather than transfusion	122	69.3
Contact by the researcher for specific permission to use all of the blood for research	51	29.0
Don't know	3	1.7
	176	100.0

TABLE 8

Of the three consents presented, which would you prefer if some of the blood you donated would be used for research?

Response	Number	Percent
General statement on card	19	51.4
Specific statement about research	14	37.8
Verbal contact with researcher	4	10.8
	37	100.0

(Did not remember statement on card about research—13)

TABLE 9

Of the three consents presented, which would you prefer if all of the blood you donated would be used for research?

Response	Number	Percent
General statement on card	18	48.6
Specific statement about research	14	37.8
Verbal contact with researcher	5	13.5
	37	99.9

(Did not remember statement on card about research—13)

TABLE 10

If there were a general statement on the consent card that there was a possibility that a very small amount of your blood donation would be used for laboratory research, would you be as likely to donate blood?

Response	Number	Percent
Definitely yes	150	75.0
Probably yes	37	18.5
Don't know	6	3.0
Probably not	6	3.0
Definitely not	1	.5
	200	100.0

TABLE 11

If there were a general statement on the card that there was a possibility your blood would all be used for research, would you be as likely to donate blood?

Response	Number	Percent
Definitely yes	108	54.0
Probably yes	53	26.5
Don't know	10	5.0
Probably not	21	10.5
Definitely not	8	4.0
	200	100.0

TABLE 12

If any of the blood you donated would be used for laboratory research, would you want to know for what research the blood would be used?

Response	Number	Percent
Definitely yes	59	29.5
Probably yes	44	22.0
Don't know	4	2.0
Probably not	52	26.0
Definitely not	41	20.5
	200	100.0

The authors are grateful to Mr. Benjamin Weinberg, Blood Bank Supervisor, and Mr. George Gonzalez, Blood Donor Recruiter at the blood bank in which the research was conducted.

CHAPTER THIRTEEN

Limits on the Right to Privacy: The Ethics of Record Searches and Other Uses of Private Materials

Some research designs pose a problem of privacy. The problem usually arises when researchers want to use existing material such as medical records, research data collected for other studies, or left-over blood, urine, or other human matter. Medical record searches provide a good example of the privacy problems raised, but the same analysis could apply to any of the other areas. Since medical records contain vast amounts of important medical data, searching them is very tempting to researchers, especially social scientists and epidemiologists. Searching them also raises problems for those concerned about access to confidential information.

A Case

Professors Samuel Lementz and Gertrude Rawlings of the Department of Social Medicine of Eastern Medical School have for many years been concerned about the spread of venereal disease in their city. They have seen rates of venereal diseases rise rapidly. They have seen medical complications and socio-psychological trauma.

They propose to launch a comprehensive study of the epidemiological patterns of venereal disease within their community. The study will take place in two phases. In phase one the researchers propose to go to the medical records of all confirmed venereal-disease cases within their hospital over the past ten years and, using the medical records, which contain detailed data about the family as well as the individual patient, construct a social-psychological profile of patients at high risk. The researchers have distinguished careers in epidemiological research. Although most of their work has been on the study of more traditional infectious diseases, they have no reason to doubt that the sophisticated methodology they use, for which they have gained such well-deserved reputation, will yield impor-

169

tant information about the profiles of persons at risk for venereal disease. . . .

Phase two of the study will involve a further search of the hospital records, this time extending the search to all records in the hospital within the past ten years. Using those records they will test the hypothesis that patients who fit the profile of being at high risk for venereal disease have gynecological or genito-urinary tract problems consistent with venereal disease. From these data they hope to accomplish two things: (1) estimate the extent of undiagnosed venereal disease within their community and (2) describe a "venereal disease profile" that will be taught to the clinical staff so they will be particularly alert to screen for venereally transmitted disease in the patients fitting the profile.

In order to assure confidentiality, no record will be made that in any way identifies the subjects whose records will be searched.

The proposed research, which is based on a composite of record-search cases I have been involved in over several years, is surely pursuing important research objectives. If done by highly competent researchers using methods and statistical tests of high quality, it could surely produce important information. Yet critics have raised a number of questions about this kind of record search. They have complained that it constitutes a potentially serious invasion of privacy. Civil-liberties proponents have insisted that, as a matter of principle, medical records are private, that the patient is the only one with authority to release information.

The defenders of the research have been outraged at the pettiness of appealing to principle at a time when there is a serious disease problem in the community and sick people are going untreated. They argue that there is no risk to the persons whose records will be searched. In fact, it is conceivable that some of them will someday benefit from the study by having diseases diagnosed that would otherwise have gone undetected. Since the names of those whose records will be searched will not even be recorded, there is no risk that the subject's sexual behaviors or any other potentially embarrassing information about them could ever be revealed.

Thus the core problem in the ethics of privacy is determining when, if ever, the pursuit of knowledge justifiably overrides privacy. The solution will depend in part on whether one really believes there are ethical duties and rights not resting directly on consequences.[1] Since we are arguing about whether it is ethically right to search the records, it is important to have some understanding of what is at stake. Over and over again those who defend the practice of searching records without subject consent or further justification reveal that for them it is the consequences that count. If, however, one recognizes that what is just or right or what one has a right to is not *necessarily* identical to that which produces the best consequences, a very different conclusion about record searches is reached. Defenders of record searches may want to defend consequentialism; many social scientists and some physicians do. (That is probably why they so readily belittle the right of privacy and the defenders of rights more generally.) But most of the Judeo-Christian tradition, our founding fathers, our legal system, and the overall view taken by the DHHS in their regulations on the protection of human subjects as well as many researchers are on my side. They believe rights are morally relevant even if honoring them does not produce the best consequences. My right to vote cannot be sacrificed simply because the society would be better off if I could not vote. The DHHS regulations are a result of that agency's commitment to protect the welfare *and the rights* of subjects, even if certain consequentialists do not grasp the legitimacy of this concern.[2] This all suggests that a right like the right to privacy may be limited, but not simply by expedient consequences.

What is the nature of this right to privacy, then, and what are its limits? Surprisingly, my formulation of the nature of the right and the nature of its limits can be taken verbatim from the text of a critic of the right of privacy, to which this essay was originally a response. E. L. Pattullo, Director of the Center for the Behavioral Sciences at Harvard University, and a critic of appeals to privacy at the expense of scientific knowledge, says with regard to research that "research subjects . . . have good reason to expect that they should not find themselves involved in unanticipated and objectionable ways."[3] This is a nicely formulated claim not limited by mere consequences. The "should," if taken as an "ought," is merely the reciprocal of a rights claim: That researchers should not involve subjects in unanticipated and objectionable ways means, I take it, that subjects have the right not to be involved in unanticipated and objectionable ways.

The "and" in Pattullo's formulation may make him more protective of the right of privacy than I would want to be. Does he mean that for a researcher to be justified in invading privacy it must be both anticipated and unobjectionable, or only one or the other? He may mean both anticipated and unobjectionable, or only one or the other. He may mean both conditions have to be met for the invasion to be justified; I think, depending on what he means, I might be satisfied with only one or the other.

What is needed is a systematic position on the grounds for placing limits on the right of privacy. I see two plausible limits: consent and just claims of others with due process. If the subject consents (i.e., anticipates and agrees to provide the useful data), then surely privacy may be invaded. In fact, we may not even want to refer to such use of information as an "invasion." If the subject does not consent, but the matter is of extreme societal urgency and ample due process has been provided, then that also may provide a justified limit on the right of privacy. Data use may therefore be unobjectionable even if unanticipated.

Let us test these twin justifications for obtaining private information by the examples Pattullo uses (two of which were taken from an earlier article of mine): reanalysis of existing data, display of surgically removed human organs, and review of psychiatric records. It could plausibly be argued that in none of these examples is any "harm" done to the subjects. In some cases, especially review of psychiatric records, real old-fashioned physical or economic harm may result, but let that be for now. I want to deal only with the cases where no harm can be anticipated. I am convinced that if subjects consented to others obtaining private information no one would have any serious problem with researcher access. I also suspect (as opposed to know) that in certain cases it would be reasonable for people to object to the proposed invasion or at least object to having the invasion take place without their consent. For example, the display of surgically removed sexual organs might be quite offensive to some people even if their names are not attached.

Some researchers say at this point that if they were the potential subjects of these studies, they would not object to these cases of making public what was previously private. Yet the fact that they would not object is irrelevant. This simply shows that researchers uniquely uncommitted to the right of privacy have different instincts about privacy than other people.

Record searches, reanalysis of existing data banks, and research use of remaindered tissues pose more of a problem. If subjects are not asked, there is no way for them to "anticipate" that they might be involved in any way. I believe, however, that many reasonable people would consent, if asked, to ordinary instances of such use of data. Some reasonable people, however, might object for various reasons. This suggests some consent process is in order. The vast majority who would consent might give a blank-check (or uninformed) consent in advance to ordinary uses of records or data in data banks. I certainly would in some circumstances. Some IRBs use blanket consent for such record studies. These consents are included as part of standard admissions forms to hospitals and other facilities that assemble records or data banks. The subject is asked to consent to have his or her records used without further contact. The subjects can "anticipate" their involvement and give an approval that is relatively uniformed in general, but nevertheless adequately informed for their purposes. Surely Pattullo would not object to giving subjects enough information so that they can anticipate their involvement. Whether subjects who object to blanket consents should be permitted to get services of that institution though refusing blanket consent probably depends on the nature of the institution. Institutions that are devoted primarily to generating research data and to which persons do not have a general right of access are the kinds of institutions that might justifiably refuse to provide services if patients refuse to sign such consents. A medical research center such as the National Institutes of Health Clinical Center would be one example. A private social-science research firm whose purpose was to generate data banks for research purposes would be another. On the other hand, institutions to which there is a general right of access, such as a city hospital, would surely not be permitted to exclude persons solely because they refused to sign a blanket consent for use of their records for research. A college psychology department might exclude students from research projects on grounds of refusal to sign a blanket consent, but it could not exclude such refusers from psychology courses. In any case commitments made by the potential subject and by the institution should normally govern access to records, remaindered tissue, blood, and so forth.

There are two problems with blanket consents, however. First, all may reasonably object to certain highly unusual uses of the data, and second, in some cases even getting the blanket consent is procedurally difficult.

Virtually all reasonable people would object to one kind of data use even when the use is harmless. This is the case whenever potential subjects would object to the purpose of the research. A consent process is complete only if it includes information about the purpose of the research. Both old and new DHHS regulations require this.[4] Presumably the reason the DHHS requires information about the purpose is that some people, in rare cases, may object to the purpose of the study. Examples of these rare instances include studies done to relate race to IQ or blood type, to develop strategies to promote abortion, to develop a theoretical foundation for biological warfare, or to gather data useful for a particular political perspective. The fact that they originally consented when data were collected for some other study with another purpose says nothing about whether they would have consented to having the data used for the new purpose.

Since upon reflection many reasonable people probably would not want to sign a blanket consent for literally any use (including uses for purposes of which they disapprove), at least one IRB has adopted the policy that blanket consents should be used to authorize "anticipated" use of records only in cases where, in the judgment of the IRB, it is implausible that any subjects would have objections related to the special nature of the project. (This means IRBs should review all such uses even when no individualized consent is planned, in order to determine that reasonable people would not object to the purpose or any other special features of the study.) The blanket consent can then include the statement that the IRB will review all uses to determine that subjects are not likely to disapprove of the research done under the blanket consent.

In rare instances, however, it seems obvious that the potential subjects would not object, but blanket consent cannot be relied upon—because the researcher wants to use old data files generated before the blanket-consent process was in place. Furthermore, it may be extremely difficult or impossible to get explicit consent for the use of these data. The subjects may have moved, died, or become too ill to consent. If blanket consent is impossible and explicit consent is extremely difficult, then possibly IRBs could consider a "constructed consent."

Researchers never get "fully" informed consent; to do so would be impossible. There is an infinite amount of information that could be transmitted. Researchers are expected only to transmit what reasonable people would want to know. It is conceivable that for some populations and some studies reasonable people would want to know absolutely nothing (including the fact that the study is being conducted). If empirically that were the case, then adequate information would be conveyed if nothing were said. A consent is constructed on the grounds that the subjects have been told all they would want to know. If use of data on this basis were widely publicized, then subjects might be said to be able to anticipate it.

The burden of proof is on the researcher either to get the consent (explicit or blanket) or to determine that reasonable people would not object to having their tissues or records used for the proposed purpose without being asked. That can be determined best empirically, by asking surrogate subjects drawn from the same population whether they would object. That seems the most accurate strategy. I and others have proposed and actually done such sampling in the past.[5] Alternatively, IRBs can try to guess at whether subjects would object. Maybe some IRBs are skillful enough to know their subjects' views and can "read" them without actual tests. Since IRBs have views on the relationship of the value of knowledge and the right of privacy that are probably not the same as the subjects', such "reading" will be risky, however.

My position is that the use of such data is "anticipated" and therefore legitimate when the subjects have consented or it is reasonable to conclude that they would not object to the use without their more explicit consent. That is Pattullo's principle watered down, but given flesh. It is watered down because anticipation alone justifies the invasion. It is given flesh by the recognition that there are good grounds why people might object even to harmless invasions.

The case of epidemiologists who want to search medical records to determine the profile of subjects at high risk for venereal disease provides an interesting case where the presumption of patient approval is problematic. The first line of analysis is one of questioning whether subjects are in any way at risk. Most defenders of the use of confidential information for research purposes concede that such use is acceptable only when subjects are not at risk. They maintain, however, that in record searches and other uses of existing data such as left-over specimens, subjects could not possibly be at risk.

The first way in which subjects in the venereal disease study could potentially be at risk is if they are still users of the hospital facilities where the information might someday be used. Although in a record search patients are not subject to any physical or psychological risk from the data collection, they might be subject to the consequences of the study. They might, for example, be in the group fitting the high-risk profile and be stereotyped by future clinicians as being at special risk for venereal disease. If the clinician knew that the patient had been a long-term patient at the facility and knew that the patient fit the high-risk profile that was constructed based on the data from these patients, the patient might be associated particularly closely with the results of the study. One strategy for avoiding this problem is to collect data from records of persons who no longer could use the service in question. Using older records would decrease the likelihood that subjects would still be using the hospital in question. It might also yield less timely results. Even so, using older records would still not eliminate the problem completely. Using the records of deceased patients would be the only way to completely eliminate this risk. In other studies—e.g., a study of successful suicide attempts—by the very nature of the study, the subjects could never themselves be affected by the results of the study.

The second area of potential risk is that of confidentiality violation. The researchers in this case have confronted this problem by insisting that identifying information not be retained. That may not completely eliminate the confidentiality violation risk, however. Sometimes data reveal a great deal without disclosing specific identifiers. If, for example, the researchers found that ninety-nine percent of the single Hispanic females using the clinic had engaged in what is normally thought to be a stigmatizing practice, a great deal is revealed without collecting identifiers. Even without these risks, the procedure of avoiding the collection of identifiers assumes that the confidentiality risk is one of having private information revealed beyond the researchers. What, however, if the researchers themselves know personally some of the patients whose files are being searched? What if some subjects object to strangers, even strangers who are researchers, seeing private information about their sexual histories? In either case, privacy would have been violated in ways potentially disturbing to the patients even though information did not pass beyond the researchers.

Finally, if blanket consent is to be used to justify searching the records for the venereal disease study or if consent is to be constructed on the grounds that subjects would not reasonably object, the IRB needs to consider whether subjects would plausibly object to the purposes of the study even if they were not at risk for either harm or for objectionable confidentiality violation. In this case, the IRB would need to ask whether any subjects would reasonably object to the project of constructing a profile of patients at high risk for venereal disease and making it available to clinicians so they can be alert for screening patients potentially at high risk. The question of whether subjects have objections to the purpose of the research is one that can only be answered empirically, using methods such as the use of lay surrogates. It seems likely, however, that some significant fraction of the potential subjects would be uneasy with this project and the stereotyping it could produce. Any person whose records are used for this study is contributing to a project that will lead to having clinicians viewing certain patients as at high risk for venereal disease. It is likely that they will extend the stereotype further, viewing such patients as promiscuous or sexually loose. If a patient wanted to contribute to the project that would generate data upon which such stereotypes might be constructed, I would not object. If the patient objected, however, I would understand. I do not think the use of a blanket consent or a constructed consent is warranted in this case.

But defenders of research use of records and other existing data are likely to ask, "Shouldn't access be acceptable in those cases where the study is still of crucial importance to society, even if the subjects refuse to consent or it can be ascertained that they would object to the use of the data without consent?" Venereal disease, for example, is a critical problem, and the welfare of others is at stake. This is a situation that requires the second justification of invasion of privacy. It is possible that other rights (not just other values) may justify overriding privacy. Rights to justice, freedom, and even to life may be at stake and override privacy rights. Such basic rights even justify military conscription, one of the most fundamental invasions of one's freedom imaginable. Here, one's privacy as well as other rights are severely limited in comparison to those rights enjoyed as a civilian. In the context of this debate I have no objection to even this fundamental invasion of privacy provided the criterion of due process is met. By that I mean that there must be public debate over the justification for overriding privacy and other rights in order to justify conscription of research subjects just as there is for military conscription; there must be an orderly procedure for societal decision making leading to the conclusion that other basic rights take precedence. Constitutional requirements must be satisfied, not merely the standards of researchers, the researcher's community, or the IRB. If it is decided by due process that an invasion of records is necessary for research purposes (as it might be for certain public-health purposes), certainly the right of privacy must be overridden. Subjects must be conscripted in order to serve other conflicting ethical requirements. This means that if a researcher is correct in his or her assessment of the importance of the invasion of privacy, the mere finding with due process that it is morally unobjectionable (because other basic rights require it) is sufficient to justify the access to the data even if it is unanticipated by the subject and even if no consent can be obtained or approval constructed.

Privacy then it seems is not so sacred after all. It can be breached whenever it is anticipated approvingly by the subject or whenever with due process it is decided that preservation of other basic rights or needs require it even when consent would have been refused. Do defenders of the use of existing data favor a policy that would compromise the right of privacy even more? Would they use records in cases when subjects refuse consent, when subjects would not approve without consent, and simultaneously society has not determined that the objective is so important that basic rights require it? Or would they limit invasions of privacy to the two justifications I have developed? If they would so limit them, they must join me in questioning the new DHHS guidelines that would permit invasions of privacy even when these criteria are not met.[6]

A case can be made for limiting the right of privacy. Doing so requires arguments about consent and justifiable overriding of privacy based on due process. Doing so also requires testing the limits of privacy by the standards of real subjects and other real laypeople, not just opinions of researchers that they would not mind having their privacy invaded and diatribe about the good consequences of limiting privacy.

PART
V

Special Research Contexts

CHAPTER FOURTEEN

"Experimental" Pregnancy: The Ethical Complexities of Experimentation with Oral Contraceptives

Sometimes ethical problems arise in human-subjects research that are not so much systematic problems of research design and subject recruitment as problems specific to particular research contexts. Examples of these include exposure of women to the risks of pregnancy from studying contraceptives, the testing of experimental contraceptives on adolescents who probably cannot be treated as consenting adults, research on brain-dead children, experiments where the expected outcomes are so attractive that the real risks may be to control groups, and experiments in treating cancer patients. Though in each of these cases there arise some basic problems of ethical theory addressed in part II and some of the special research-design and subject-recruitment problems addressed in part IV, the unique nature of these experiments suggests that they deserve separate attention. In the next several chapters, these special research contexts will be examined.

The first problematic study, the study of the side effects of oral contraceptives, was the first specific research project I had analyzed publicly. In some ways its problems were the most obvious; its abuse the most blatant. Yet it poses, in its most stark form, the conflict between reasoning that attempts to produce benefit to society as a whole and the more patient-centered reasoning that insists on adequate information for patients and adequate protection of patients regardless of the benefits to the broader society of the proposed research.

The study is an older one. The work was published in 1971. Quite possibly the more rigorous federal regulations and the more sophisticated review boards in place today would not have permitted this study to be done. Nevertheless, 1971 is not the dark ages. It is several years after the publication of Henry Beecher's famous exposé of ethical problems in biomedical

178

research.[1] It is several years after the Department of Health, Education, and Welfare began developing guidelines for the protection of human subjects. It was studies such as this one that made clear that we had, and perhaps still have, a long way to go to assure that subjects have their rights and welfare protected adequately.

Whether it achieved its original purpose or not, this experiment with birth-control pills proved conclusively that (a) placebos do not prevent pregnancy, and (b) the issues raised in biomedical research are complex and sometimes vexing.[2] The experiment, conducted mostly upon poor, multiparous, Mexican-American women who had come to a San Antonio clinic for contraceptives, raises numerous medical, ethical, and social questions.

According to Dr. Joseph Goldzieher of the Southwest Foundation for Research and Education, who conducted the experiment, its purpose was to find out whether some of the reported side effects of oral contraceptives were physiological or psychological. In a double-blind experiment, 76 of the women received dummy pills while another group got various hormone contraceptives. All had come, not to assist in research, but to prevent further pregnancies. None were told they were receiving placebos, or even that they were participating in research, but they *were* instructed to use a standard, prescription vaginal cream or foam in addition to the oral contraceptive "until it was certain that they were using an effective pill."[3]

The results: the women on placebos had many of the same side effects—nervousness, depression, breast tenderness, and headaches—as those on The Pill.[4] But 6 of the 76 women on placebos became pregnant. The results of this study were reported to the American Fertility Society, first described in *Medical World News* and later published in the scholarly journal *Fertility and Sterility*.

Some of the more obvious ethical questions were raised in the *Medical World News* report. Dr. Christopher Tietze of the Population Council was quoted as saying that "No responsible investigator would take it upon himself to expose women seeking protection to the risk of pregnancy by ostensibly giving them . . . mere glucose, or at best some vitamins."[5] Besides this rather obvious breach of ethics, there are other difficulties involved in the study that are also of great importance.

Importance of the research. It is clear that at least some people thought this research was important. Certainly there is considerable confusion about the side effects of oral contraceptives. It would indeed be helpful to know more. More than that, many unwanted pregnancies and a statistically measurable number of maternal deaths could be prevented if it could be shown that side effects were a figment of the imagination and because of this women returned to The Pill.

On the other hand, one critic was quoted as saying that "the thing that bothers me most about this study is that the results weren't worth it."[6] It needs to be determined who should decide whether the results of an experimental procedure are even potentially "worth it." Given that scientists may have more than a typical commitment to the value of knowledge, it is questionable that they should be the ones to decide. One prevalent view is that government policy makers are needed. An argument may also be made that experimental subjects should have a say in whether the research in question is important insofar as they should be told of the purpose of the study before providing consent to be a subject.

Institutional controls and review procedures. This experiment raises serious questions about the levels of control over experimental procedure. Informed consent is a classical ethical norm of experimentation on human subjects. Anyone who thinks he can get "fully" informed consent is naive (all we ever strive for is a reasonably informed subject), but there was not even a semblance of informed consent in this experiment. Why could patient subjects not be told, as one critic suggests, that there is a placebo group in the experimental design?[7] If patients then knowledgeably refuse to participate the message should be clear.

In many research institutions and funding agencies review procedures are now established. Yet the procedures in effect at the Southwest Foundation for Research and Education are unknown. The study was funded by Syntex Labs, a manufacturer of oral contraceptives, and the federal government's Agency for International Development, an agency with primary interests in an area other than biomedical research. It is important to know what Syntex's interest was in this project, and what their review and control procedures consisted of. Would the experiment have been approved for funding by the National Institutes of Health? If not, then perhaps the moral is that if one wants to conduct questionable research he or she should seek out research facilities and funding where fewer questions will be asked. Further, one must establish that a study funded in large part by a drug manufacturer can be expected to be as impartial as one funded which does not have a vested interest in the outcome.

Publication. Responsibility for ethically acceptable research goes beyond funder, institution, and researcher. It is a questionable practice for publishers to accept reports of research where consent procedures are not clearly specified. By providing a public forum for the research, a publication or a learned society shares responsibility for the research. Thus it is unclear whether *Medical World News* and *Fertility and Sterility* should have transmitted the findings of this work to the nation's medical community. *Medical World News*, however, at least also provided a critical discussion of the ethics of the study. It is questionable nonetheless whether members of the scientific community—such as the American Fertility Society and the journal *Fertility and Sterility*—should publish studies that fail to offer thoroughly explained consent procedures. We are well beyond the day when professional journals and professional societies can plead value-free scientific objectivity. Whether or not they finally decide to participate in the research by providing a public forum, professional journals and societies cannot avoid facing the hard ethical questions.

Design of the experiment. Besides the obvious failure to provide informed consent concerning the placebo, there were other difficulties as well. The four other groups in the experimental design received either high-estrogen sequential, high-estrogen combination, low-estrogen combination, or chlormadinone acetate. Of these, sequentials were well known to have substantially higher failure rates. High-estrogen combinations were being used less frequently because of often documented higher incidence of side effects. Chlormadinone acetate was a research progestin, which had since been banned from all further human investigation because of reported side effects observed in beagles.[8] The experimental design, even without the placebo group, raises all of the same questions about consent and review. If it is wrong to expose women unknowingly to pregnancy risk from placebos, it is questionable whether it is right to expose them to smaller, but already documented risks from sequentials.

The research design included the use of vaginal cream to give additional contraceptive protection. Leaving aside the questions raised by the use of an admittedly poor back-up contraceptive agent, does not the introduction of the vaginal cream necessarily convey to the patient that she is getting something other than routine oral contraceptive agents? In Dr. Goldzieher's own words vaginal cream "just doesn't work all that well."[9]

Abortion as a back-up. Dr. Goldzieher is quoted as saying that "we could have aborted them if the abortion statute here in Texas weren't in limbo right now."[10] (An appeal of the Texas law was before the Supreme Court at that time.) Certainly he does not mean that the law's being in limbo put greater restrictions on him than a firmly established anti-abortion law would.

But there is an even more fundamental ethical question raised with the suggestion that abortion should be a back-up for pregnancies induced for the good of scientific experiment in the face of the explicitly expressed wishes of the individual woman not to become pregnant. Many persons—perhaps those involved as subjects—believe that abortion is not such a trivial procedure that it can be casually introduced in this way. Further, one should at least consider the physical and psychological consequences to the woman, if not to the conceptus. Since it could reasonably be predicted that several of the women who conceived in the experiment would be morally opposed to abortion under these circumstances, this would have to be taken into account if back-up abortion were incorporated into the research design.

The researcher's responsibility. A researcher conducting experiments on human beings must assume responsibility for the harmful effects of the experimental procedure on the subjects. Were the experimenters and funders of the research in this case willing to make that ultimate commitment? If so, was it really the case that no abortions were available to the women who conceived? This seems unlikely in light of the millions of abortions being performed yearly throughout the world even before the 1973 Supreme Court decision legalizing abortion. Even more fundamentally, are the researchers and the funders of the research now prepared to provide financial and other support for the products of their experiment? The subjects seem to have a just claim not only for full support for the children produced, but for the psychological and social burdens placed on them as parents. The researcher should be prepared to offer such assistance. Legal aid should be available for the parents who may have to bring suit.

The use of clinic patients. This case makes clear that the ethical implications of biomedical research are usually social and rarely merely personal. The subjects for the experiment were "almost all of them Mexican-American and poor."[11] It is interesting to consider whether the same results would be obtained among upper-middle class women—say, male researchers' wives. The fact that *clinic* patients, that is, people too poor to pay for medical care— were the subjects for so much of the biomedical research conducted raises questions concerning the fairness of research practices.

Deterioration of trust. Finally, the clinical and the scientific community also have a stake in the ethical execution of each individual research project. Even if this particular act of deception could be defended on the basis of the utility of the knowledge to be gained, what is its effect upon the clinical institution involved, upon clinical institutions generally, and upon the scientists who are attempting to carry out morally acceptable research? Trust is a central value in the patient-physician relationship. Each such violation challenges that trust in a very realistic way. Each researcher, when evaluating his or her experimental design, has an obligation to protect that trust and confidence along with his or her primary obligation to protect the interests and well-being of the subject.

The case of the placebo for contraception raises even more ethical questions than are at first apparent. The question now is: What steps are now being taken to prepare the scientific community and the society at large to cope with these questions and protect themselves against potential future ethical abuses?

CHAPTER FIFTEEN

Contraception Research on Teenagers: Beyond Consent to Treatment

When contraceptive or other medical technologies are developed and tested on adults, it cannot be assumed that the effects will be the same when used on children or adolescents. After the initial trials on adults, a judgment must be made that the risks to the minor are justified by the potential benefits to the patient or at least that the net risks to the minor are minimal. At that point the initial tests for most drugs on minors can be authorized with the permission of parents or guardians. In certain special contexts, however, parental permission is problematic.

In an essay entitled "Can Teenagers Participate in Research without Parental Consent?" to which this chapter was originally written as a response, Yale lawyer Angela Holder suggested that there are several contexts in which parental consent (or permission, which is the term now usually applied) would not be necessary. Holder points out that some adolescents are considered emancipated minors. They are living essentially on their own without parental supervision or control. She points out that married minors, minors in military service, and most minors who are self-supporting and living away from home are now considered emancipated. She also describes the group referred to as "mature minors." They have demonstrated that they are capable of understanding the nature of the decisions to be made and, therefore, as with emancipated minors, are capable of giving an informed consent. In both cases, parental permission is probably unnecessary either legally or ethically.

In a number of special cases minors who are neither emancipated nor certified mature are given the authority to assent to treatment without parental permission. Statutory authorization permits minors to assent to certain specified medical procedures without parental permission—procedures such as contraceptive and abortion services, and treatment for venereal disease, drug abuse, and alcoholism. In addition, some states permit adolescents to consent to any medical or surgical care without parental involvement after the age of, say, 15 or 16.[1] Holder implies that in any of these areas where treatment on minors is permitted by statute without parental permission *research* on treatment would also be permitted without such permission.

On some points I have no disagreement with Holder. Emancipated minors can consent to treatment or research interventions, as can any competent adult. Mature minors are able to consent although there is no way to be sure that a minor is "mature" unless a researcher has obtained a prior judicial determination. There may be extreme cases of medical therapy where this course would be worth pursuing, but it is hard to think of cases where judicial review would be appropriate merely to determine that a teenager is mature enough to understand and give an informed, voluntary consent for *research* without parental involvement.

My contacts with several IRBs suggest that this kind of research is more common than one might at first believe. The problem arises when teenagers are obtaining medical treatment under the special provisions of state laws permitting them to be treated without parental permission. Since these services often represent some of the most sensitive and important medical encounters, it is understandable that researchers may want to conduct studies using these adolescents as both patients and subjects. Since the laws normally provide for these treatments without parental involvement precisely because they are so sensitive, obtaining parental permission for the adolescent to participate in the research component also raises problems.

This is the background for proposals to permit minors to assent to research in these areas. The National Commission for the Protection of Human Subjects, for example, commented that "if parental permission were required for research about such conditions, it would be difficult to develop improved methods of prevention and therapy that meet the special needs of adolescents."[2] The implication is that assent from minors alone without parental permission is justified in cases where the law permits them to assent to treatment without parental permission. I think that is an erroneous conclusion.

There is a crucial difference in justification in the cases of treatment of teenagers and research involving teenagers. I believe there are two possible reasons for the laws permitting minors to assent to certain treatment without parental permission. First, in all the situations a requirement of parental permission would almost certainly deter the minor from getting necessary medical attention. Parents may reasonably prefer to waive their right to give permission for medical treatment in these special situations because it would be in the minor's best interest to get treatment rather than to avoid it. While not all parents may take this position, it seems likely that the vast majority would do so. Second, even if some individual parents do not want to waive their right to serve their children's interests, the state may conclude that these treatments are so much in the minors' interests that they should be rendered independent of parental permission.

Of the two explanations, the first seems the most plausible. There is no claim that the minor is competent to consent to these special treatments, or that he or she is emancipated or even mature, in the sense the law uses the term. It is simply a special case in which physician paternalism justifiably replaces parental paternalism.

It is easy to see why the laws should not be extended to allow adolescents to assent to medical research without parental permission, even in the areas dealt with by specific statutes. Such a leap would permit a minor who is not capable of consenting to assent to a procedure without the participation of his or her legal guardian in a situation in which the benefits to the adolescent (alone) do not justify the minor's participation. Recall that, if we are speaking of randomized clinical trials, the research procedures are being undertaken in order to determine whether the net benefits of the new treatment exceed those of the standard treatment. It is research because we do not know whether the net benefits exceed the net benefits of standard treatment. One cannot hold this and, at the same time, argue that the experimental intervention is of critical importance to the minor's welfare in comparison with standard treatment.

Consider a related example. A researcher wants to study the blood levels of a contraceptive in first-time adolescent pill-users. The researcher may believe that first-time adolescent users are a unique population, and so cannot use other subject groups, such as adults. Furthermore, since these subjects will never again be first-time users, they will in no way benefit from the research. Of course, the normal moral requirements for research must be met, including the conducting of the study first on adults who can consent. Some would argue that because the adolecents can legally assent to getting the pills, they should also be permitted to assent to having blood drawn for the purposes of study to benefit other, future users.

But if this view is justified, it cannot be because reasonable parents would believe that the study is so much in their child's interest that they should concur in the waiving of their right to give permission. It must be the very strange reason that the Commission gave in Recommendation 8: that important research would be jeopardized if a fuller permission-gathering process were required.[3] But that is to assume that consent, assents, and permissions may be waived simply because the research would be hurt. That is a crass appeal to social utility at the expense of individual rights. That move, however, might justify the Nazi experiments. Of course I am not suggesting that either Holder or the National Commission would condone such research, but they have not shown adequately what the limits are to their justification of waiving valid consent on utility grounds.

Utility alone has never justified waiving consent in the United States. DHHS regulations require, as they should, not only the finding of a favorable benefit-harm ratio so that society's interests are served but, independently, a legally adequate consent as well as other requirements.[4] There is a provision for waiving consent, but stringent requirements must be met including that the risk to the subjects will be minimal, that the research could not practicably be carried out without the waiver or alteration, and that the subjects will be provided with additional pertinent information after participation. A fourth requirement is that the research may not "adversely affect the rights and welfare of the subjects."[5] If one of the rights of subjects is a right to information that they would want to know in order to decide to participate in the study, then, unless it can be demonstrated that the withheld information would not be desired by the subjects, no waivers can ever take place.

I have no objection to a general reformulation of the age of majority or even the age of majority for the specific purpose of giving consent to research interventions that are not of potential benefit to the subject. The age when a person can give an informed and free consent is an empirical question. If empirical evidence shows that this age should be lowered, I would not object. However, the age when an adolescent is really able to give informed and voluntary consent should not be changed merely on the grounds that it is difficult to ask parental permission. I also have no objection to application of mature minor laws, provided we have some due process to assure that the minor is mature.

Even if this argument is not accepted, there must be severe limits placed on an IRB's right to waive parental permission in these cases. The Commission proposed rather elaborate safeguards including an appropriate mechanism for protecting the children who will participate as subjects. It suggested that a clinic nurse or physician not involved in the research explain the nature and the purpose of the research to prospective subjects, emphasizing that participation in the research is unrelated to provision of care. Another proposed alternative is the use of a surrogate parent.

Another limit is implied in the Commission recommendations, although it is not spelled out specifically. Holder points out that an IRB probably would not authorize research on adolescents without parental permission if there "were more than minimal risk of physical harm." The Commission never specified this qualification. If they had addressed the problem, they certainly would concur in some limit on the risk. They did in fact recommend that routine research on minors without prospect of direct benefit can only involve "a minor increase over minimal risk" even if parental permission is obtained.[6] Certainly their recommendations would not permit adolescents themselves to assent to greater risk without parental involvement. The Commission would appear, therefore, to limit research with only adolescent assent to situations with no more than minor increase over minimal risk. In fact they might prudently have limited it to no increase over minimal risk.

Furthermore, the Commission did not limit the risks to physical ones as Holder does.[7] Some of the studies may involve greater psychological risks than physical ones—studies of guilt over a previously conducted abortion, for example. Even the drawing of bloods from adolescents in the context of statutorily authorized medical treatments offers some unexpected risks. In the case of the adolescent receiving contraceptives, if blood were drawn for a study, how would the young woman explain the needle marks to her parents? Should researchers or subjects be left by themselves to anticipate such risks? Should they be excluded simply because they are not physical risks?

As Holder points out, the DHHS regulations incorporate some of the Commission's views. They do not adopt the Commission's Recommendation 8 in full, however. The proposed regulations say, "If the IRB determines that a research protocol is designed for conditions or for a subject population for which parental or guardian permission is not a reasonable requirement to protect the subjects (for example, neglected or abused children), it may waive the consent requirements . . . provided an appropriate mechanism for protecting the children who will participate as subjects in the research is substituted, and provided further that the waiver is not inconsistent with federal state or local law."[8]

Holder assumes that drafters of the regulations limited their examples to neglected or abused children while intending that the waiver apply to other cases as well. Admittedly the regulations are silent and ambiguous, but I think the dropping of all the Commission's references to treatments authorized without parental permission was purposeful. How could parental permission be seen as not a reasonable requirement to protect the subjects in these cases? Parental permission for the minor (or minimally above minor) risks for these interventions without direct therapeutic intent is just as protective in these cases as in other cases where parental permission would be required. The adolescents are in no way put in jeopardy because they, by definition, do not benefit from the research the way they would from the related treatment interventions. It may make sense to seek alternative protection for abused or neglected children, but not for children subject to special medical treatment statutes. In those cases there is no reason to assume the parents could not protect their children's interest in research interventions lacking the prospect of direct benefit.

The case for waiving parental permission is particularly weak in this situation because most of the research can be done rather adequately without the waiver. Presumably many groups of adolescents would be available to the researcher: emancipated minors, adolescents who have reached the age of majority, and minors who are receiving the medical care with parental knowledge who could obtain the routine parental permission.

It might be argued that this excludes a group from the population being studied: the immature, unemancipated minor who is getting medical care without parental permission. At the very least the study should first be conducted on all the groups where consent, assent, and permissions can be obtained without complication. Only then should research on this special group who cannot or will not get parental permission be considered. Even then the decision for the IRB to authorize the research without parental permission and with only the assent of the minor (not the consent that is informed and voluntary) is problematic. The only justification is that it is useful to society to do so. I think that step is unnecessary and unjustified.

CHAPTER SIXTEEN

Research on the Brain-Dead: A Special Case of Research on "Non-Consentables"

Researchers proposed to test the effectiveness of the esophageal obturator airway (EOA), a device used to facilitate artificial respiration on children 2–14 years old. The EOA is currently in standard use for non-hospitalized patients over 15 years.

According to Ronald A. Carson, Jaime L. Frias, and Richard J. Melker, who originally published the case study to which this chapter was originally prepared as a commentary:

> The EOA is a curved plastic tube—similar in appearance to an endotracheal tube. At one end it is mounted on a face mask, which is rimmed by a soft cuff; when pressed lightly against the face, this cuff creates an airtight seal. The other end of the tube is closed; just before this end there is an inflatable balloon.
>
> In use, the tube is passed blindly into the esophagus, the mask is seated on the face, and the balloon on the tube is inflated. Because the esophageal end of the tube is closed and the balloon blocks the esophagus, air or oxygen blown into the tube escapes through ports located in that section of the tube that resides in the throat and enters the trachea to inflate the lungs. Blockage of the esophagus prevents distention of the stomach with air during artificial ventilation; it also prevents regurgitation of stomach contents which, under these conditions, would be very dangerous.[1]

The researchers did not want to expose the first children upon whom this EPA would be tested to any risks. They therefore chose a special group of subjects. The children used as subjects in the study had met the accepted standards of brain death, though the brain-death standard had not been legally adopted in the state in which this protocol was proposed. The parents and physician of each subject had made the decision to terminate artificial life supports.

Informed consent was obtained from the parent or guardian of each child before each subject was randomly assigned to one of two groups, one of which would be ventilated first through an EOA and then through an endotracheal tube and the other would undergo the identical procedure in reverse order.

Carson, Frias, and Melker suggested that one ethical issue that they believed pertinent to the EOA protocol was determining "appropriate criteria for determining that a person has died (currently considered unproblematic due to the widespread adoption of the 'brain death' criteria)."[2] They proceed in their evaluation to assume that there is no question that it is appropriate to assume the patients in question are dead. This assumption is evident in their formulation of what they believe is a key ethical question the IRB must address, namely, "Is it at all appropriate to interject, between the pronouncement of death and the final leavetaking, an experimental procedure?"[3]

If the potential subjects are considered dead, they are, in effect, respiring cadavers. The requirements of the Uniform Anatomical Gift Act as passed in the state where the research is being conducted would apply. Newly dead who have not previously objected can be used for therapy, transplant, or research with the permission of the next of kin. With that permission, I see no moral objections to the study.

Yet it is not obvious that the subjects proposed for the research should be considered dead using brain criteria as the basis of that judgment. While some 25 states had established in law that brain criteria could be used for death pronouncement at the time of this study, the state in which this research was proposed was not one of them. I think it is risky morally (probably legally as well) to presume that the legal standard for pronouncing death can be changed by an individual medical practitioner, a researcher, or an IRB. It seems to me safer for the IRB to err on the side of assuming that the old common-law tradition still applies until the state formally changes its position. Although I believe the law should be changed, heart and lung criteria should be used for determining whether these particular children are to be viewed as alive or dead. Yet even if the IRB decides to consider the subjects as living children (albeit without brain function), it is not clear that the IRB's decisions would necessarily differ. The subjects would not stand to benefit from the research intervention to test the EOA regardless of whether they are considered alive or dead.

If the children were considered alive, it is possible that they might still be used as research subjects. Some ethicists analyzing the problem have concluded that "non-consentables," that is, those who lack the capacity to consent, cannot be used as research subjects except when the research intervention would, on balance, be of potential benefit to them. Others, however, including the National Commission for the Protection of Human Subjects of Biomedical and Behavioral Research[4] and the writers of the current DHHS regulations,[5] have concluded that such use of non-consentables is acceptable if certain strict criteria are met. Among these are that the permission of the parent be obtained and that the research intervention expose the subject to only minimal risk (or possible minor increments above minimal risk).

The testing of the EOA in children with significant survival potential probably is above minimal risk or even above the vague level called minor increments above minimal risk. Thus it could not be tested on such children if they could not be expected to benefit proportionally. Some would conclude that this means that the EOA should not be tested even in the children who are proposed for this study. Others, however, argue that for those particular children the EOA may, in certain circumstances, be of no risk whatsoever. That would at least be the case in situations where, having dead brains, they could not experience pain or discomfort and where the parents had exercised their parental responsibility to decide that, given their child's medical condition, treatment should be withdrawn as unfitting.

It seems clear, given the Quinlan, Saikewicz, and many other legal cases as well as the long tradition of medical ethics, that parents have not only the right but the responsibility to decide whether continued treatment would benefit a child who has no hope of recovery of any brain function.[6] In such situations some parents will decide that the most morally appropriate course is to remove any further treatment so that loving care can most appropriately be substituted.

Can parents ever at this point consent to have their children be used as subjects for an experimental testing of a device that can do no harm to their child, but can do no good either? Although there is a risk that some parents might abuse the responsibility, I see no reason why parents, properly screened and counseled, should be prohibited from making this moral judgment. If this is the case, then parental consent would be required, but would, if the other conditions are met, make the research acceptable.

One of the issues at stake in the design of this protocol was whether to return the children to respirators following the study. Carson, Frias, and Melker state in their evaluation of this protocol that "if the child is determined to be in irreversible coma, to be dead, and *then* engaged as a research subject, there is neither logic nor merit in returning the newly dead subject to the respirator at the end of the study."[7] With that I certainly agree, but this would also be the case if the parents had exercised their responsibility to stop treatment on the living child on the grounds that it was useless or unfitting. Then it would also be inappropriate to return the child to the respirator after the research. If it is justifiable to do the research on the dying child, it is certainly justifiable to continue the course of withholding interventions designed to prolong the dying process. I do not see any moral or criminal liability sanctioned by such a decision.

The IRB might have considered two other alternatives. First, consider the position of those who object to conducting the research on children who are appropriately being allowed to die based on parental judgment of the child's best interest, but who accept research done on the newly dead when death is based on the brain criteria. For them the research could be conducted without the legal and ethical problems if it were transferred to a state that has adopted a definition of death based on brain criteria. I would not object to conducting this research under the provisions of the Uniform Anatomical Gift Act in such a state.

Second, presumably some children are currently being treated who potentially might benefit from the use of the esophageal obturator airway. The entire problem of the ethics of research interventions unrelated to possible therapeutic benefit could be avoided if the device were tested on these children. It is an empirical problem whether the potential risk to them would be sufficiently great that this could not be done acceptably. If there were a group who would surely die without the EOA, but might live with it, they would be the best group of patient/subjects. Experimentation on non-consentables who can stand to benefit from the intervention is generally preferable morally to interventions on those subjects who cannot. If, for technical reasons of unacceptable risk, that were not possible, I would prefer to transfer the research to a state that has adopted a brain-oriented definition of death. If that were not possible I would, if I were a member of the IRB, urge the conceptualization of the case as one of research on dying children rather than one in which the researchers and the IRB would, without due process, rewrite the state laws on the definition of death.

There is a final question for the IRB. What is the extent of the IRB's responsibility to assure that the parents are approached humanely and can tolerate the invasion of their privacy at a time of deep personal family tragedy?

Carson, Frias, and Melker summarized the IRB's position on this question as follows:

> It would be essential that the experiment honor the mechanically sustained body and the parents' memory of the person who was (is, still—death is not "the end" for the parent) their child. What is likely to matter above all will be the attitude and tone of voice of the investigator seeking the parents' permission. If he bears in mind that he is a supplicant, that he is asking for something precious, and incorporates that knowledge in the asking, there is no reason not to ask. The decision is the parents'. So reasoned the IRB in approving this project.[8]

When the regulations under which IRBs operate call for assurance that appropriate informed consent is obtained, I believe they generate an obligation on the IRB to examine not only the quality of the information transmitted, but also its psychological impact. In extreme cases, such as this one, the one being asked to consent (or give permission) may simply be so traumatized that consent is impossible. The IRB did make these considerations part of its responsibility and should be commended for it.

IRBs facing similar situations may have techniques available to help them assess the humaneness as well as the technical quality of the consent process. In research studying the bereavement process of parents who have lost children to sudden infant death syndrome (SIDS), some researchers have constituted an advisory panel of parents who at some previous time have experienced such a loss. The IRB asking questions about how traumatic the consent process would be for bereaving parents might make use of such a panel. The standard seems clear. The parents should be told of those things and only those things that parents similarly situated would have wanted to be told. If enough information cannot be transmitted on that basis to get adequate consent, then the research simply cannot be done. The input of laypeople situated as similarly as possible as the eventual subjects is essential. The IRB may learn from them that research intervention in such situations would have been so offensive and so traumatic that it was morally intolerable. On the other hand, they may learn that parents could handle the request quite well.

The task of the IRB in this case was enormous. It required knowledge of complex state law, the philosophical debate over the definition of death, the ethical controversy over the acceptability of using non-consentables as research subjects, the technical risks of conducting such tests on children who might actually benefit from them, the psychology of the consent process, and parental evaluations of the humaneness of research interventions at a time of personal tragedy. Because it is not unusual for the typical protocol to be at least as complex ethically and conceptually as is this EOA protocol, a highly sensitive analysis, such as the one which the IRB provided in this case study, is required before one can be assured that a particular study is justified.

CHAPTER SEVENTEEN

Risk-Taking in Cancer Chemotherapy

This chapter is a case study of one institutional review board's lengthy debate over a proposed pilot study involving chemotherapy for a small-cell carcinoma of the lung, a particularly serious and intractable tumor. The IRB served at a major urban teaching hospital. Federal regulations require the local IRB to determine whether "risks to subjects are reasonable in relation to anticipated benefits, if any, to the subjects. . . ."[1] They provide little guidance, however, for helping the IRB make that often extremely subjective determination. The chemotherapy protocol provided an exercise in risk assessment.

THE PROTOCOL

As one of a long series of studies examining the effectiveness of several chemotherapeutic agents, the researcher proposed to administer in high doses the five most active agents available for the chemotherapy of the disease. He wanted to determine the toxicity, make an initial estimate of the activity of the combination, and determine whether such an intensive regimen would be suitable for multicenter cooperative group trials.

The five drugs to be studied were cyclophosphamide, adriamycin, VP-16-213, vincristine, and methotrexate. The toxicities of the first four drugs were known to researchers and clinicians in the field and to several members of the IRB. These risks, which the IRB had evaluated in many previous protocols, included nausea, vomiting, myelosuppression, stomatitis, alopecia, and cardiomyopathy. While the toxicities are unpleasant and sometimes serious, the patients who would be subjects of the study were all seriously ill with a type of tumor that has proved particularly resistant to standard therapies.

194

Methotrexate, the fifth agent, can also have serious side effects (my-elosuppression, stomatitis, occasional hepatitis, nephrotoxicity, and neurotoxicity), particularly when given in high doses. The proposed study called for a relatively high dose ($1.0gm/M^2$ i.v.), but it would be followed by the administration of leucovorin, an agent known to neutralize the toxicity of the methotrexate and permit administration of the methotrexate in much higher doses.

The five-drug combination was to be administered repeatedly in twenty-one day cycles, with the methotrexate given on the fifteenth day. The leucovorin was to be administered intravenously exactly twenty-four hours after the methotrexate and then given by mouth for three days. Complete histories and physical examinations for each patient were to precede the study and to be repeated throughout the study. Patients were to be screened for admission to the study; they had to meet appropriate medical standards and give informed consent.

The members began the process of reviewing the protocol on risk-benefit grounds. The original debate concerned the risk-benefit ratio of the five-drug regimen, especially the high-dose methotrexate component. In addition, the question of the mode of administration of the leucovorin rescue agent was raised. The patients were to be treated on an outpatient basis. They would receive the intravenous leucovorin at the hospital. Serum methotrexate levels would be monitored, but unless they were too high, the remaining leucovorin would be taken by the patient at home.

Some members of the IRB became concerned about the risk of this mode of administration. They felt that it would be safer for the patient if all the leucovorin were administered while the patient was hospitalized. They pointed out that these patients might well have difficulty remembering to take the leucovorin. The effects of the disease, combined with the side effects of the chemotherapeutic agents, might make them confused or disoriented. Furthermore, such patients might become depressed. The psychological set might cause them to forget their medication. Some patients might even purposely choose to omit the doses, with serious, potentially even fatal, results. Some members held that the acceptability and efficacy of the five-drug regimen should first be studied under optimum conditions, that is, in a hospital. Then, if that proved out, one might consider the additional problem of outpatient administration of the leucovorin. The debate that took place over the risk of the protocol even on an inpatient basis paralleled many that take place regularly in IRBs. The controversy over the outpatient administration of leucovorin, however, was rather unusual. It also revealed how different members of the group were arguing from different basic principles.

THREE POINTS OF VIEW

Three general points of view emerged over the course of the debate of the proposal for outpatient administration of the leucovorin.

1. *Protecting the patient from harm.* One group of IRB members

focused on protecting the patient from harm. They became very concerned not only about the toxicity of the five-drug regimen, but also about the added risk of administering the leucovorin in the proposed manner. They felt that the risk to the patients could be decreased by treating them as inpatients during the course of the leucovorin administration. It was pointed out that an important task of the IRB was to protect human subjects. In fact, current federal regulations require that the IRB determine that the risks to the subject are so outweighed by the sum of the benefit to the subject and the importance of the knowledge to be gained as to warrant a decision to allow the subject to accept the risks. Some members felt this could be accomplished by hospitalizing the patients. The core moral commitment of the IRB members who took this point of view seemed to be that the task of the committee was to protect patients. For some, this meant refusing to approve even a marginal, but strictly speaking therapeutically unnecessary, increase in risk that would come from administering the drug on an outpatient basis.

The risk of purposeful refusal to take the leucovorin rescue agent as a way of hastening death was a risk that seemed to be in a special moral category. Independent of the question of the ethics of suicide—a question the IRB felt it need not debate—some members felt that it was unacceptable for the protocol to offer the patient a way of hastening death. It is often argued that the physician's moral obligation is to prolong life. While it is increasingly recognized that it is sometimes inappropriate to struggle too long against an inevitable death, using medical skills and resources to provide ways to hasten death might well be morally quite another matter.

It seems clear that the researcher would not begin the chemotherapeutic regimen with a patient if he did not believe that the proposed therapy was appropriate. Presumably the patient would make a similar decision. The patient, of course, might initiate the treatment with therapeutic intentions but decide at some later point to take advantage of the remarkable set of circumstances to end his or her life. All this points to a special problem of the possibility that the protocol could be used to hasten death.

The IRB members could have classified this as an additional harm. This would have required the assumption that the purposeful refusal to take the rescue agent would really be a harm for the patient on balance. For those focusing on protecting the patient's real interest, there was particular concern that a patient not act precipitously in a way that would not really be in his or her interest. One member observed that ending one's life in a hospital would require persistence, steadfastness of purpose, and an unshakable conviction that death is desired. On an outpatient basis, however, the patient may be possessed by a passing whim, a transient depression, or a momentary madness and could do the deed before anyone could stop or even argue with him or her. From the standpoint of avoiding this kind of harm to the patient, inpatient administration would be far preferable. Alternatively, a member could take the position that, independent of whether refusal should count as a benefit or a harm, it is simply morally unacceptable to use medical skills and resources in a way that could lead to the purposeful hastening of a patient's death.

Members of the IRB who took this first general position insisted that for the protocol to be approved there would have to be significant adjustments. Arrangements would have to be made to protect the patients from the risk of failure to take the leucovorin properly and from other harms that might come to patients if they were treated on an outpatient basis. The members seemed to prefer administration of the drug on an inpatient basis, but also discussed among themselves intermediate possibilities such as administration of the drug by a visiting nurse.

2. *Social concerns.* A second general point of view focused more on the potential harms that would come from the inpatient administration of the leucovorin and how those harms compared to the potential harms of home administration. It was pointed out that the resources of the clinical center were limited. Some raised the concern that requiring hospitalization of these patients for three days out of every twenty-one might tax the facilities beyond their capacity. It might mean that other patients who could have used those facilities would be excluded or would have to be treated elsewhere. The concern was not only for the high economic costs of inpatient treatment but for the limited resources of personnel and facilities.

Also the researcher was interested in developing a mode of therapy that could be used widely. It was his belief that even if in-hospital administration could be arranged at this institution it would not generally be feasible. Seen from the perspective of the interests of other members of the society, the problem is not one of simply exposing these patients to marginal additional risks of home treatment, but one of deciding when a marginal risk to one group of patients is worth taking in order to provide benefits or at least save costs to the society.

Certainly not every conceivable benefit to society would justify taking risks with patients. The charge to the IRB is to determine whether these particular risks, especially the marginal risks of home administration of the leucovorin, are justified by the combined value to the patient and others. Those who defended the home administration had to consider not only the potential benefits to others of the home administration but also the severity of the risks to the patient. The researcher, in a communication to the committee, emphasized that he recognized that some of the patients might be unable to follow the prescribed antidote regimen. His team planned to exclude patients they felt to be unreliable, because they could not be reached quickly by phone should their methotrexate levels at twenty-four hours be elevated, because they were alcoholics or drug addicts, or because they were so sick that travel back and forth to the hospital for frequent evaluation would be extraordinarily difficult. He also pointed out that his team had developed a system by which patients can be brought back to the center rapidly should there be any question of increased toxicity.

Further, as evidence that outpatient administration can be safe, he referred to an experience he had treating five patients on this protocol at another center (not under the jurisdiction of this IRB). These patients had experienced no toxicity. He also pointed out that at another institution 243 patients have been treated with weekly highdose methotrexate with rescue, in doses three to ten times as high as those he proposed to use. In that study, the incidence of severe toxicity for each dose of methotrexate was less than 3 percent, and was less than 20 percent overall. There was one treatment-related death, a patient who deliberately did not take any of his leucovorin. The researcher reported that at the other institution the investigators found the outpatient mode of administration successful and convenient. The members of the IRB who agreed with the researcher agreed that, in this case, the risks to the patient were justified.

3. *Freedom of choice.* A third general point of view focused on the importance of the patient's convenience, a subjective variable. Different patients are likely to evaluate the inconvenience of returning to the hospital differently. For some, taking the drug at home, with the risks involved, may be viewed as too traumatic despite the convenience. For others, however, the thought of being hospitalized for three days out of every twenty-one, especially when one is extremely ill with a condition that might well be fatal soon, is unacceptable.

Some members of the IRB took the position that risks and benefits were not the only critical moral variable in this case. For them, freedom of choice or patient autonomy was also significant. From this general standpoint, the subjects should have the right to accept the risk of home administration as long as the risk is made clear in the consent process and appropriate safeguards are provided (such as adequate plans for rapid return of the patient to the hospital if it becomes necessary). For at least one of the IRB members, who placed particular emphasis on this point of view, patient self-determination rather than risks and benefits to either patient or society was the important consideration. This approach avoids the more difficult ethical problem of deciding under what conditions risk to a patient is justified by potential benefits to others. At least for those patients who choose to have the leucovorin at home, the problem of scarce resources is avoided.

Several problems remain for those who hold this position, however. First, what about the patients who would prefer hospital administration of the rescue agent? If they were a small number, perhaps the clinical facility could accommodate them. Even then, they would be accommodated at some costs to others, but the cost might be bearable under certain circumstances. What, however, if the number were large? It would be hard to predict without some informal questioning of potential subjects. It would seem morally awkward to accept only those patients who exercised free choice to take the drug at home, while excluding those who wanted it administered in the somewhat safer hospital setting.

The self-determination principle also creates problems for those who feel that even if individuals should have the right to self-determination, that right cannot require others to cooperate with their choices. Some IRB members felt it was wrong for them, as agents of the institution, to collaborate in permitting a patient to take a risk that the IRB members personally thought was unacceptable. Some took a similar stand, not generally about the extra risk of home administration, but about the possible purposeful refusal to take leucovorin. For those who stand firmly for the principle of self-determination, the right to refuse treatment remains a crucial legal and ethical right. For those who emphasize protection of the interests of the patient or society, however, including government officials and private citizens, these considerations may justify overriding patient self-determination. In any case, the right of the physician and the institution not to participate in research they consider morally offensive must remain a crucial moral issue for the IRB.

BASIC ETHICAL PRINCIPLES

The three points of view that seemed to emerge in the debate over the case seem to represent three basic ethical principles held by members of society, including those who happen to be members of IRBs. The first position commits the physician to doing what he or she thinks will benefit the patient. It emphasizes the welfare of the patient, recognizing that the interests of others may be left unfulfilled. This is a position that has dominated traditional medical ethics from the Hippocratic oath to the present and is one of the concerns reflected in governmental regulations[2] and the Declaration of Helsinki.[3]

The second position is more decisively social in its orientation. It emphasizes the necessity of permitting patients to take certain risks, in order to produce what its adherents consider to be greater benefits. While not dominant in traditional professional codes such as the Hippocratic oath or Percival's Code, this commitment is incorporated in many other public documents such as the Nuremberg Code,[4] and in U.S. regulation.[5] It is also present in the World Medical Association's Declaration of Helsinki, which reflects the medical profession's recognition that permitting so-called "non-therapeutic clinical research" is not consistent with the position that only the patient's interests are morally relevant.[6]

The third position, that focusing on liberty and self-determination, leads to the conclusion that benefits of either kind—to the patient or to society—are not decisive. This commitment to self-determination as the basis of judgment has its origin in sources quite different from the other two positions, and is quite incompatible with the traditions behind them, such as the Hippocratic oath. It is a commitment arising from the modern, liberal Western culture, and has penetrated Anglo-American law, for example, in Justice Schroeder's opinion in the famous *Natanson* case on informed consent, when he says that "Anglo-American law starts with the premise of thoroughgoing self-determination."[7] In its most extreme form it leads to the conclusion that any competent individual should be able to do anything to himself that he wants (take a drug, have his leg amputated if he has a certain kind of fetish, refuse therapy for himself, etc.), provided only that the anticipated consequences are limited to the individual himself.

It is understandable that researchers, IRB members, and others who struggled with this case over the months of debate reached different conclusions. In addition to all the possible misunderstandings of fact and all the breakdowns in communication that can take place when individuals representing different disciplines attempt to understand protocols as complex as this one, the individuals involved in the review of the protocol emphasized different ethical commitments as well. Since no IRB member is likely to opt simplistically for any of the three principles, the decision of the IRB will depend upon how the different members balance the competing principles as well as how they weigh the empirical data before them. In this case a majority voted against permitting the outpatient administration of the leucovorin.

In the process a number of questions remain. What would have been the outcome at another institution where there might be a somewhat different emphasis in presenting the facts of the case and where IRB members might hold a somewhat different mix of ethical principles? Given the months of effort that went into the reviewing of this protocol—the memos back and forth between committee and researcher and the appearance of the researcher at a committee meeting to discuss the protocol—given the scores of hours it took to develop the discussion even to this point, what would have been the result in another institution where such conscientious efforts by committee and researcher might not be present? Was there more that could have been done even in this case? Were the IRB members adequately aware of the researcher's willingness to hospitalize patients who would choose to be hospitalized? Was the researcher aware that the IRB might have been willing to consider compromises such as supervised home administration of the leucovorin? The federal regulation requiring and accepting the balancing of risks to the patient by benefits to the society as well as the patient is controversial on its face. The application of the regulation, requiring as it does subtle judgments by individual IRB members coming to the problem from very different traditions, is even more difficult.

CHAPTER EIGHTEEN

The Ethics of Research Involving Radiation

In some ways research protocols involving exposure of subjects to radiation present the same problems for IRB members as those encountered in other research proposals. Risks must be compared with benefits to the subject and others; subjects must be reasonably informed; the usual rights of the subject must be protected; and subjects must be selected equitably. At a practical level, however, proposals involving potential radiation risk raise unique, perplexing issues. Radiation exposure places directly at risk in addition to consenting subjects, other human beings—bystanders, lab personnel, and even future generations. Not only are potential effects not known, but most IRB members have very little understanding of the mechanisms of action of radiation and even the basic concepts underlying its effects. Because the field of radiation itself is politically and socially controversial, IRB members necessarily find themselves participating in a larger social debate.

RISK ASSESSMENT

One major problem facing IRBs is risk assessment. It can honestly be said of most research involving radiation that there is no conclusive evidence that exposures called for in the protocol are harmful. Still the overwhelming consensus is that some risk, however small, remains and must be considered. Under the older DHEW regulations the decision about whether any risk was present made a significant difference to IRBs (because review was triggered by federal regulations only when risk was present).[1] Current DHHS regulations, however, make no such distinction.[2] IRB review is called for in protocols involving radiation exposure whether or not subjects are deemed to be at risk. While certain categories of research are exempt from review and other categories can be given expedited review, any research governed by DHHS regulations involving the exposure of subjects to radiation, no matter how little, certainly does not fall into either of those classes.

In assessing risks of harm and comparing them to potential benefits IRBs face several problems. First, the IRB is normally considering an extremely small probability of harms, many of which, however, if they occur, will be very substantial. Moreover, the IRB is often working with what is at best a rough estimate, often based on an extrapolation from exposures in a very different setting at much higher radiation levels. There is theoretical disagreement over the legitimacy of the extrapolation. In such a situation substantial disagreement over the degree of the risk is expected.

Because of the highly technical nature of the data, IRBs will probably have to rely on the testimony of experts, often one or at most two IRB members or consultants. Yet even the experts differ greatly in deciding what the risk level is, whether it is legitimate to extrapolate data, and how serious the harms will be if they do occur. The contribution of a single expert source will have to be evaluated by other IRB members, even those with little or no medical training. If, for example, those who have chosen to make nuclear physics and radiation medicine their careers have personalities that make them either particularly fearful or particularly unconcerned about the effects of radiation, other IRB members will have to take those influences into account in incorporating their view in the IRB's deliberation. This same problem exists, of course, when the IRB uses any expert consultant. It is a logically necessary part of the process of selecting from an infinite array of potential observations those that are considered important or significant. It is thus a necessary part of the scientific enterprise and not in any sense a flaw or deficiency in the expert's ability. Still in an area where the basic science and the conceptual apparatus is so alien to most IRB members and the subject matter is socially and politically controversial, the risk of this kind of problem is particularly great.

When the type and probability of harms is established, the IRB will then have to determine how bad those harms would be if they occurred and how those harms compare to the value of the knowledge potentially gained. The National Council on Radiation Protection and Measurements refers to "permissible dose standards."[3] While IRBs have occasionally used occupational and therapeutic permissible dose standards for comparative purposes, say, five rads of radiation per year, it does not follow that the person should also be permitted to be so exposed at that level for research purposes. "Permissible dose standards" are, after all, merely value judgments about how risk of harm compares to the potential benefits from work or therapy. They are not directly relevant to research.

Much of the debate over determining these traditional kinds of risk may simply be preliminary to the question of how the subject is to be told of the risk. If subjects knowledgeably consent to these risks, once described properly, much of the IRB's concern will have been met. Radiation research, however, involves a second kind of risk—risk to other parties, to offspring of subjects, family members, and even bystanders.

The risk to bystanders and postnatal family members from low-level radiation used in most research is sufficiently low that it is often ignored by IRBs and probably appropriately so. Certain research, however, involves much larger exposures where risks to others may have to be taken into account as they are in almost no other research protocols. The clearest example is the debate over the nuclear-powered artificial heart. The federal government's Artificial Heart Technology Assessment Panel had reservations over the risk to spouses of the radiation exposure that might come from a nuclear-powered heart.[4] An IRB reviewing a protocol to test a nuclear-powered heart would have to determine whether the risks to another party were justified as well as the risks to the subject.

Technically this extends the IRB's mandate. It is charged with assessing the risks to the subject and comparing them with the anticipated benefits to the subject as well as the value of the knowledge to be gained. Clearly, however, explicit risks to other parties must also be on the IRB's agenda. Alternatively one might argue that any third party put at such risk should automatically be classified as a subject, be asked to consent, be monitored and so forth. The level of radiation to third parties that would trigger this review is, as yet, undetermined.

The more ordinary problem of risk assessment in radiation research is risk to others in the form of risk to fetuses or even to future offspring through genetic damage to gametes. This risk is well-known and guarded against by having more rigorous standards for exposure for pregnant women and requirements from gonadal shields for radiation exposure when possible. That the additional risk is known, however, does not resolve the ethical question of whether such a risk is acceptable. Exposure of fetuses to such a risk could reasonably be considered an experiment on the fetus without consent. If so, it would have to be justified by the same techniques that are used for studies exposing other non-consentables to experimental risk.

Debate on the subject is heated, ranging from the conservative position that no risk is permitted to a non-consentable for the purposes of gaining scientific knowledge (that is the position attributed to many in Britain and, in the United States, to spokespersons such as Paul Ramsey) to the liberal, utilitarian view that aggregate net benefit justifies any fetal risk. Richard McCormick, occupying a cautious middle position, argues that limited exposure of non-consentables to risk is acceptable, provided certain stringent safeguards are met, including a requirement that the risk be minimal. The ground for this position is that there are certain things every member of the human community owes to others simply by being a member of that community, even if that person is unable to consent; he or she would or should consent if that were possible.[5] Radiation studies often then become, in effect, research protocols involving more than one subject. One subject normally can consent to risks involved and is asked to. Others occasionally could consent, but until now have not normally been thought of as subjects. Still others—fetuses and future offspring—in principle cannot consent to the risk to which they are subject.

CONSENT

The second major issue raised by radiation research is that of consent. The subjects, whoever they are, must be told the procedures used and the reasonably foreseeable risks. The problem is determining what procedures and what risks to disclose. On the one hand, it could be said the researchers wish to inject a substance that in the dose administered has never been shown to do any harm to humans. On the other hand, it could be said, equally truthfully, that the subject is to be exposed to radiation that is known to be related to cancer and genetic changes in those exposed and their offspring.

The problem is largely one of how uncertainty should be conveyed to subjects. There are two basic questions: Does the researcher say anything about the radiation and, if so, what?

While some have argued that the lack of any clear evidence proving harm from small-dose radiation justifies nondisclosure of the presence of radiation, most now conclude that some explanation of the use of radioactive materials is called for, no matter how small the dosage. Current legal and moral opinion seems to be converging around the standard that subjects should be told those things they reasonably would want to know or would find material to their decision to participate in the research. This, for example, was the standard articulated by the National Commission for the Protection of Human Subjects when it spoke of informed consent being based on information that the subjects may reasonably be expected to desire in considering whether or not to participate.[6] This is a conclusion rooted in commitment to the ethical principle of respect for persons although, as a side effect, it may also be a policy that promotes good consequences. It is critical to realize that this standard of informed consent, however, is not being adopted because it will help subjects or anyone else. It is derived from what the courts call a thorough-going commitment to the principle of self-determination.

If that is the standard, in determining what information about radiation should be disclosed, one needs to discover what it is reasonable to expect subjects would want to be told. That is an empirical question subject to testing by IRBs in local institutions. Given the highly emotional status of the subject of radiation today, however, it seems clear that at least some reasonable subjects, probably a substantial percentage of them, would want to be told of a research exposure to radiation, no matter how small. At least the burden should be on the researcher and the IRB to demonstrate that subjects would not be interested in knowing about such an exposure. Legal as well as moral jeopardy might result from failure to inform about such a demonstration.

If, however, some information is to be transmitted, then how much? The critical question seems to be how to transmit information when there is substantial uncertainty. The uncertainty is somewhat unusual in radiation research. It is not like the uncertainty occurring in all pharmacological research in which some totally unanticipated harmful effect may occur. Many are concerned about specific, serious anticipated harms. On the other hand, these concerns are not based on one or two cases reported in experimental as opposed to control groups. For those problems additional short-term study will clarify the relationship. With low-dose radiation the concern is over very long-term effects, effects that in principle cannot be verified in ongoing research because of the complex causal sequence and long time frame. Some other research presents the same problem, the uncertainty with mutagens in chemical plants, for example, but it is particularly acute in radiation studies.

The concern is over a suspicion well grounded in theory, but a suspicion incapable of confirmation or refutation within the time frame of the study. Should sociological facts such as the existence of "widespread feelings among scientists and others that an exposure may be harmful" count as one kind of fact that ought to be disclosed to subjects? If the criterion were whether the information would be beneficial or harmful to the subject on balance, the answer seems difficult to determine. Some subjects might be helped by the information, calmed by the realization that researchers are being open in conveying their uncertainty; others may be disturbed, fearing that researchers do not know enough about what they are doing. It seems fair to say that if benefit and harm to the subject is the criterion, different IRB members will reach different conclusions and probably within any institution some subjects will be helped on balance by the disclosure while others will be upset.

If the criterion is what it is reasonable for subjects to want to know in order to determine whether to participate in the study, then disclosure becomes a matter of rights. Subjects who would want to know would have their right to self-determination violated by nondisclosure while those who would not want the information would merely be upset, and they have the option of minimizing that harm by dropping out of the study. It seems clear that at least some reasonable subjects would want to know of the uncertainty. If they have a right to that information based on the principle of respect for persons, withholding it constitutes a violation of their rights.

What may not be clear is how rational it is for a person to want to know of uncertainty. Some decisions should be made only when there is substantial evidence supporting the decision. The decision to publish the findings of a study would be an example. Some decisions, however, must be made in the absence of firm evidence. Deciding to participate in a research protocol involving radiation exposure would be an example. For some, who are risk-averse, knowledge that the effects of radiation are uncertain could be critical in deciding rationally that they do not want to participate. Others, less risk-averse, may rationally decide to participate, but may still find it worth knowing of the uncertainty.

For both types it is meaningful to be told about the concern that even low levels of radiation may be harmful and that no exposure is widely believed to be safer. This has led IRBs in at least two major American research institutions to adopt the strategy of conveying in one way or another to subjects as part of the consent process not only the fact that radiation exposure is involved in the research, but that there is concern that some risk, though probably small, may be involved. One institution, after telling the subject that the amount of radiation is small, says, "These amounts of radiation may be potentially harmful, but because they are so small, the risks are very difficult to measure." The other contains in its standard consent form wording for small-dose radiation exposure the statement: "Every person receives a certain amount of natural radiation each day. While it is widely believed that any amount of additional radiation, however small, is less desirable than no additional radiation, the amount of radiation exposure is this procedure is less than. . . ." The statement is then completed with a comparison comparable to those recommended by Naomi Alazraki, chief radiologist, at Nuclear Medicine Service, VA Medical Center, Salt Lake City, such as "that of a routine chest x-ray."[7]

These two IRBs have faced the problem of how to convey realistically to subjects the fact that radiation exposure is involved and that some finite risk of harm is present, even though on balance many, implicitly including the members of the IRB, consider it a risk worth taking.

Somehow IRBs must struggle to determine estimated risks of harm in an area where not enough is known and typical IRB members know very little. After they have satisfied themselves that they have some appreciation of the type and probability of harm relatively untainted by the biases for or against of their expert sources, they must determine how bad the harms would be if they occur, how good the benefits of the study will be if they occur, and whether the risks to third parties are justified, either by making them additional consenting subjects or by techniques available for making them unconsenting subjects. Finally, the IRB must develop some method of conveying to the subject realistically the uncertainty that exists in the entire area.

PART
VI

*Emerging Themes and
Controversies*

CHAPTER NINETEEN

A Summing Up

A great deal has happened since Thomas Percival, the father of Anglo-American professional medical ethics, condescended to support experimenting on the poor provided "the gentlemen of the faculty" were consulted first. Medical research now takes place in a world far different from that of William Beaumont, whose studies on the gastric physiology of Alexis St. Martin were possible by forcing St. Martin to agree to a lifetime of indentured servitude in exchange for treating a life-threatening gunshot wound.

As great as the change has been between these nineteenth-century views of the ethics of research and the climate for research in the mid-twentieth century, in some ways that change may be no greater than the one taking place between the one on the horizon and the atmosphere in the early medical regulations of the 1960s and 1970s.

The internal professional debate has received a mighty stimulus from federal regulators and a Congress distressed by such revelations as those of the Tuskegee Syphilis Study, the Jewish Chronic Disease Hospital study in which live cancer cells were injected into unknowing patients, and Dr. Goldzieher's study in which he gave placebos for oral contraceptives. Together, they have gone a long way toward eliminating some of the most egregious risks of physical harms to patients. It is much harder today for a journalist to write an exposé of unethical research or for a teacher of medical ethics to find ethical outrages among published research articles. That is good.

At the same time, we have all become more sophisticated. Researchers have become more sophisticated. Risks to subjects that they would not have thought twice about twenty years ago are now not even proposed. Investigators know that they would not get past local IRBs. Just as encouraging, the investigators themselves have developed more sophisticated consciences so that they would not be comfortable exposing subjects to such risks. The review process is more sophisticated. If an investigator, for malicious reasons or, more commonly, for reasons of good, but misguided intentions, does propose risks to subjects that are out of proportion to potential benefits, the chances are much greater that the IRB will block the study. If it does not, the administrators in the funding and review process and, ultimately, the courts are likely to object. The bureaucracy has created a climate where it does not pay to expose subjects to serious, disproportional risks. Whether that climate has also discouraged important studies that could and should be conducted ethically is still open to question.

THE PATIENT AS AN ACTIVE PARTNER

At the same time, subjects are more sophisticated. While there was a day when patients, and even healthy volunteers, would assume that investigators were the appropriate ones to decide whether new procedures should be tried and whether the potential risks to subjects were justified by potential benefits to subjects and others, today that naiveté is rapidly disappearing. Increasingly patients and healthy volunteers are realizing that investigators, even assuming they are well intentioned, have agendas that do not always coincide with theirs. Deciding that it is reasonable to participate in an investigation requires much more than determining what the potential risks and benefits are. It requires determining how serious those risks and how important the benefits are and determining whether the benefits outweigh the harms. Sometimes it even requires a debate about whether an effect is a harm or a benefit. These are all questions that do not require medical expertise to answer. In fact, having medical expertise may systematically provide distorted answers. Investigators, those who have given their lives to pursuing scientific knowledge, will predictably give answers to these kinds of questions that are atypical. We should normally expect anyone who has given his or her life to pursuing scientific knowledge to place a higher value on such knowledge than the typical subject.

Subjects are also discovering that there are important elements of the decision to participate beyond comparing risks and benefits. In addition to the ethical principle of beneficence, several other ethical principles are critical. We have emphasized autonomy and justice, but promise-keeping, truth-telling, avoiding killing, and gratitude are also often of concern. Deciding what role, if any, these other ethical principles should play in the decision to participate in research is also not a technical medical question. Some people will limit their decision to the factors of benefit and harm. Others will trade off risks and benefits with other, deontological considerations. Still others will give a priority to these other principles so that, contrary to what nineteenth-century researcher Claude Bernard said, experiments that may do good are acceptable only when they do not violate the requirements of autonomy, justice, and other ethical principles. Deciding what the relationship is among autonomy, justice, and beneficence is, once again, not a technical medical question. Moreover, there is good reason to suspect that investigators are not identical with medical laypersons in the way they relate beneficence to the principles of autonomy and justice. These are judgments that each person ought to make on his or her own based on religious, philosophical, and ethical systems of belief and value. These judgments, in turn, affect the judgment about whether it is appropriate to participate in a particular piece of research.

The result is that protecting the patient from egregious harms is important, but far from adequate. There was early progress in eliminating these most serious risks primarily because there was a substantial consensus, no matter what ethical and value positions one adopts, that such exposure is wrong. But the ethics of medical and behavioral research includes more subtle judgments as well. It requires determining whether modest benefits to society or subject justify modest risks, whether minor benefits to society justify minor risks or inconvenience to the subject when that subject cannot benefit in any direct way. It requires determining how much information must be transmitted for a consent to be adequately informed. It requires determining whether the purpose of the research is worthwhile in the subject's eyes and how altruistic the subject wants to be. All of these need to be determined based on the subject's particular beliefs and values, which are not necessarily those of the investigator, the investigator's institution, its IRB, or the funding agent. The result is a need for an active subject participation in the assessment of the research such patient (or volunteer) is in a real sense a partner, although a limited partner, in the project.

The implications of this are crucial. An active subject with his or her own beliefs and values may assess a research protocol differently from the investigator at any point in the research process. Active patients or normal volunteers may, for example, have perfectly rational reasons why they would not want to participate in a randomized clinical trial, even in cases where the investigators and their colleagues sincerely believe that there is absolutely no reason to choose one treatment arm rather than another. Patients may have different risk-aversion profiles leading them to prefer the high-risk/high-gain or low-risk/low-gain arm. They may prefer the arm that has a treatment modality or plan of hospitalization that is particularly attractive to them. They may have uniquely high fear of radiation or chemicals. They may prefer a research ward or an outpatient treatment. Any of these may be differences among the arms of a random trial crucial to the patient, but a matter of indifference for the investigators or IRB. The active patient—who is a partner in the decision-making process—will have to assess each of these variables in the light of his or her own values, which may be different from those of the investigators. When potential subjects are absolutely indifferent between two treatment arms, there is no reason why they would not permit random assignment. They are at what can be referred to as the indifference point.

That indifference point may not be the same as the indifference point for the investigators or the IRB. Investigators are ethically justified in offering research participation when the randomly assigned treatments are at or near the indifference point *in their judgment*. Subjects are justified in participating when the treatments are at or near *their* indifference point. This may mean, for example, that some patients may refuse to participate when investigators are justified in making the offer, but it may also mean that some subjects are quite happy to participate (they are truly indifferent in the case of a randomized trial) even though the investigators themselves have a preference for one arm or the other. Provided the investigators do not see such a radical difference in the treatment alternatives that it violates their consciences to make the offer, they are justified in entering or continuing a study even though they see some possible preference for one arm or the other and they can find subjects who are really indifferent or are at least willing to be altruistic enough to sacrifice their assured access to the arm they prefer.

Active subjects will want to have all the information that could reasonably be meaningful to them in deciding whether to participate. This will include not only potential risks and benefits; it will include information about the purpose of the study, the alternative ways of conducting it, who the other potential subjects could have been, and anything else that could influence their decision to participate. They may well want information even in cases where no risks at all are involved such as in record searches, in certain clandestine observation, or in the use of pathological tissues and left-over blood samples. If they are to be viewed as active partners in the research, they must know the information that would permit them to make an informed judgment about their participation.

The notion of an active patient goes even further than the decision to participate. It can include being active in the design of the research as well. The case for semi-randomization made in chapter 9 is one example. If some patients have sufficiently strong preferences for one treatment arm over another, especially if they are among the least well-off of our society, they may have a case for changing the design in order to accommodate their strong preferences for one treatment or the other. If scientific objectives are also served—as, for example, in testing the hypothesis that randomized and non-randomized patients receiving a treatment respond similarly—then cooperation between investigator and active patient has changed the design, perhaps even changed to make it better science.

The methotrexate study in which the leucovorin reversing agent can be given on either an inpatient or outpatient basis is another example where active patients as partners in research design can actually change the protocol. In that case learning that patients had a preference for outpatient treatment could permit the investigators to serve patients better without any significant cost in scientific objectives. As a fringe benefit, the study would be much cheaper, leaving research funds for other important investigations.

It is reasonable to assume that in virtually every research protocol,

patients as active partners in research design could make constructive proposals that would at least change their perceived costs and benefits of
participation. In some cases this will come at no cost to the science; it may
even improve the scientific quality. At the very least it would further the
long-term goals of science by involving patients more directly and more
enthusiastically as part of the research process rather than leaving them to
perceive themselves as outsiders, passive guinea pigs, or even victims. It is
at least good public relations and may improve the quality of science in the
long run. The case for inviting patients and normal subjects to participate
routinely in the design of research is a strong one once one recognizes the
legitimacy of their claims as respected human beings with important agendas
of their own that can be brought into harmony with those of investigators. At
the very least patients and other research subjects should routinely have the
chance to read the research protocols.

THE IMPLICATIONS FOR IRBS

This provides a new agenda for institutional review boards. It can no longer
assume that its role is simply to protect subjects from harm. That is certainly
on the agenda, but is just as certainly not the only thing. Since subjects need
to have a much richer range of information to be active participants in
research than simply to protect themselves from harm, the IRB has the task
of making sure that that information is provided. The subjects need to have
the opportunity to determine whether there are other approaches to the
investigation—outpatient leucovorin rescue from the methotrexate and certain protocols where semi-randomization would be acceptable, for example—that serve the patients' agendas while helping or at least not hurting
significantly the researchers'.

If the patient is to be an active participant, then the IRB cannot simply
substitute its intuitions about these questions for those of the patient or
normal volunteer. The IRB must acknowledge that it is not the type of body
that can justifiably assume that its positions on these crucial ethical and value
issues are random. A good case can be made that, at least for some functions
of IRBs such as determining how much information should be transmitted
and determining whether risks are worth it, the IRB should be as much like
the typical subjects as possible. Adding one or two laypersons will not be
adequate, assuming that other members of the IRB would not share the
subject perspective, and that a shift in consensus in the direction of the
majority is to be expected (the risk-shift phenomenon). However, even if by
some miracle the IRB perfectly reflected the beliefs and values of the typical
reasonable members of the society, it is not clear that those views can
justifiably be imposed on the patient. If the patient is an active partner, then
he or she needs the opportunity to participate in designing the research as
well as deciding for him or herself whether to participate in it.

Devices such as the use of lay surrogate panels can be helpful in determining what reasonable laypersons would want to know or whether they would want to know anything at all about a particular study. They at least can tell us more accurately than an IRB's intuitions whether subjects similarly situated would like to be informed of a record search or of the existence of preliminary data. They could, for example, help establish whether subjects would object to being deceived in social psychology research. There are surely some questions that, in principle, cannot be answered by individual subjects—such as whether to omit pieces of information. These can probably best and most accurately be answered by surrogate panels such as those described in chapter 12. Other choices, however, such as whether two treatment arms are sufficiently near the indifference point that randomization is acceptable, can only be answered by specific, real potential subjects. The patient-as-partner model of research involving human subjects involves the recognition that patients have much more to contribute to the research process and much more interest in decision making in research than traditional passive views of patients as the recipients of research interventions.

PROBLEMS ELIMINATED WITH THE
ACTIVE PATIENT VIEW

The model in which the patient or normal subject is an active participant will solve many of the perennial problems of human-subjects research ethics. The problem of whether the risks are too great to impose on a subject almost vanishes. The risks are never imposed on subjects, they are accepted freely by well-informed participants who had a hand in designing as well as in executing the study. The problem reduces to one of whether the researchers and institutional decision makers can, in good conscience, let informed subjects volunteer for the risks involved without violating their researchers' own consciences. That is a serious question, but not as awesome as the former burden of deciding what risk is justifiably inflicted on uninvolved, unknowing subjects.

It has the potential of solving the malpractice problem, or at least a significant part of it. Malpractice as we know it today arises from two quite different sets of events. In some cases physicians are truly negligent in performing their procedures. If the knife slips and cuts the nerve when it should not or if the investigator erroneously administers ten times the experimental chemotherapeutic agent and kills the patient, there is true negligence. Patients so injured should surely be compensated. If it happens often from the same practitioner so that we can conclude that it was not an accident, that practitioner's malpractice rates should increase to such a high level that he or she is effectively excluded from practice.

I am convinced, however, that these accidental injuries are not the real cause of most malpractice claims today. They come from a second kind of negligence: negligence in failing to encourage patient involvement. If the clinician in either research or routine practice is aware of a risk and does not inform the patient, he or she runs the risk that the uninformed patient will be justifiably angered should the statistically predictable risk occur. When it does, the patient is naturally going to seek redress for the totally unanticipated though predictable injury.

If the patient is an active partner in the decision-making process informed of all risks that reasonable persons would want to know about, then that patient can choose whether to accept the risks involved. Should the patent be the loser in the lottery and suffer the statistically unlikely untoward consequence that he or she knew about and accepted, that patient surely has no ethical claim to compensation beyond that available as part of health insurance or as part of the research facility's offer to the patient. It is reasonable that risks accepted for the good of science, for example, be covered by a promise on the part of the institution to make good where possible with medical treatment and rehabilitation when injuries occur. In fact, a rational active patient probably would not consent to research procedures if he or she were not assured of adequate care in the event of an accident. But extravagant jury awards for what amounts to the pain and anger of unanticipated injury would essentially be eliminated. An active patient consenting to the risks and protected with a reasonable remedial treatment plan should be entitled to nothing more, whether the claim arises in research or in routine clinical medicine. The malpractice problem, as a serious threat to medical professionals, would no longer be a problem if the model of the patient as partner in the medical process were realized as the most justified alternative.

The most serious problem resolved by the patient as active partner model of research is probably neither the problem of deciding how much risk to impose or the problem of malpractice. It is probably what could be called the problem of the patient as material—as research or teaching or clinical material to be manipulated as an object—either for its own good or the good of others. The traditional model of the physician-patient relationship in which the physician fulfills his Hippocratic obligation to benefit the patient regardless of whether the patient's integrity is respected has as its most fundamental flaw the dehumanization of the persons who are patients. The shift to the research context in which the welfare of the society is added to the welfare of the patient/subject does nothing to rehumanize the person who is the object of study. The model in which the patient is an active partner in the process, a knowing intelligent human being with his or her own agenda, preferences, and ideas has the most profound advantage of overcoming the indignity of the manipulative mode of the more traditional relationship. That may be the most profound advantage of the patient as partner model.

REMAINING CONTROVERSIES

The patient-as-partner model is a model of research with human subjects, not research on human objects. It will not solve all the problems of human-subjects research. It will even create new problems where none existed before. Most of the new problems, however, are problems that were finessed only because patients were so excluded from the process that their interests and their rights could be ignored. The patient-as-partner model and the reasonable-person standard of informed consent that is integral to it create enormous problems. It creates the problem of deciding what reasonable people would want to know and how to treat subjects whose views do not match the hypothetical reasonable person. It also creates the problem of preliminary data. It may well be that there are some studies that will never be able to get to the point of an adequate level of statistical confidence because reasonable persons would want to know of preliminary data trends prior to the time when enough data are generated to reach a conclusion at the precious 0.05 level. If that is a new problem generated by the patient-as-partner model, it is only because the researchers in the older model ignored their duties to their patients in order to pursue admittedly important knowledge for society's benefit. As long as patients were viewed as passive objects to be manipulated, they could get away with it. No one asked the terrible question of whether reasonable patients would want to know about the preliminary data trends. Once the question is asked, however, there is no avoiding the potential conflict. It is reasonable for investigators to want to push on to an adequate level of statistical significance, and it is reasonable for patients to want to choose the arm of the study that is producing the better preliminary data—at least in cases when the difference is one of life and death and when the data trend has developed to the point that it is nearing the desired level of significance. The ethical conflict is real. The patient-as-partner model does not solve it, but it at least does not pretend that it does not exist.

The patient-as-partner model of active patient participation in the design and execution of research creates some problems for researchers who have been able to count on existing pools of data in medical records and other confidential sources of information. This model requires asking some difficult questions such as whether reasonable persons would want to be informed that their confidential records are being searched and what the purpose of the experiment is. Since some reasonable people would not like to have the records searched, this presents a serious problem. Perhaps sometimes it will be justified for researchers by using lay surrogates to establish that reasonable persons would not object to having their records searched without their consent. Stated more carefully, surrogates could establish that reasonable subjects would want to be told nothing in order to have a consent adequately informed. That device combined with blanket, uninformed consent and, potentially, conscription of unconsenting subjects as part of a broader community decision with due process provides limits to the problem of studying existing data and specimens. It does so without the nasty reduction of the subject who generated that information to an object to be monitored without consent, involvement, or knowledge.

Probably the most serious problem advocates of the patient-as-partner model of research face is the problem of research being conducted that is not mandated by DHHS regulation to be reviewed for protection of human subjects. Currently DHHS regulations apply by law only to research funded by the Department. Since fundamental human rights—rights to have one's autonomy respected through the consent process and rights to have justice in the selection of human subjects and rights to have one's privacy protected— apply even to those persons who are subjects of studies not funded by DHHS or otherwise in the DHHS nexus, this is a serious problem. If the ethic of human-subjects research is an ethic of the patient as partner, then all research on human subjects, not just DHHS-funded research, must meet the standards outlined here.

Fortunately, most reputable research institutions apply at least the DHHS standards to all human-subjects research within their walls. The Department of Health and Human Services and the Congress have, however, missed a golden opportunity to extend the requirement as a matter of law. They could have applied it to all institutions receiving federal funds, to all institutions dealing in interstate commerce, or all institutions receiving Hill-Burton funds. It is unfortunate that they have not found some such way to assure that many of the human participants in non-DHHS research are given the same rights and protections as those who are. It is, after all, the subjects involved in non-DHHS funded studies who are probably in greater jeopardy, given the rigorous federal review process.

Fortunately, some states, such as New York, have passed laws that accomplish protecting these subjects by applying state standards (which are identical to federal standards) to all research in the state not governed by DHHS regulations. If one is worried about creeping federalism, this is an effective way to provide protection at the state level.

Closely related is the problem of research exempted from DHHS regulation. In general, research conducted in established or commonly accepted educational settings or involving the use of educational tests, research involving survey or interview or data collection procedures, or observation of public behavior (as long as subjects are unidentifiable) are all exempt. As we have seen, the regulators, apparently lapsing back into the era when only research involving real risks of harm to subjects was thought worthy of regulation, exempted this research from any required scrutiny. They exempted it in spite of the fact that real rights of subjects are involved—such as the right to consent to the purpose of the study. In doing so, they violated the notion of the patient as an active partner in the research enterprise. In fact, they created a world in which you and I can be participants in research literally without even knowing the study is being conducted. That is the ultimate in passivity, the ultimate violation of the active patient participation model. A good case can be made that no research should be conducted without any IRB review, at least expedited review. Involvement without further patient participation should take place only when there has been a blanket consent, a constructed consent, or conscription with due process, all of which provide some kind of patient participation. All studies justified through these methods need IRB review.

If the model of the patient as active partner in the research process is adopted, ethical problems will still remain. The problems of subjects who benefit and actively consent, but benefit only because they are so miserable are not solved, but a principle of justice can be appealed to begin formulating a solution. The problem of subjects who consent with adequate information to research risks that some of us consider beyond reason remains. A non-paternalistic basis for addressing this issue—an approach based on treating the investigators and their institution as ethical agents who must, based on their own conscience, decide when to participate in research—gives us a way to approach the problem. The problem remains of deciding, in the use of surrogate and other reasonable-person strategies, what percentage of persons would constitute an adequate percentage for concluding that some reasonable persons would want to know. If it is not the arbitrary five percent that I have proposed, then what is the basis for a rational defense of some other position?

All of these problems are inherent in a model for research that involves the patient and other human subjects as active partners in the research process. While they are significant, they are much more sophisticated problems than those that arose with the earlier model of subjects as passive objects who were researched upon rather than with.

The model of the patient as an active partner is one that draws research ethics and clinical medical ethics much closer together. I am more and more convinced that the model presented here—the model of the patient as active participant in a partnership governed by the ethical principles such as autonomy and justice as well as beneficence—applies equally to routine clinical medicine as well as research. Exactly the same analysis would provide guidance for treating the relationship between the clinical health professional and the layperson as a limited partnership in which individual sets of beliefs and values converge leading to decisions that are possible only when the patient is an active participating partner in the relation. That, however, is a subject for a second volume of *The Patient as Partner*.

NOTES

GOVERNMENT DOCUMENTS CITED

U.S. DEPARTMENT OF HEALTH, EDUCATION, AND WELFARE (DHEW)

"Protection of Human Subjects." *Federal Register* 39 (May 30, 1974):Pt II 18914–18920.

The Institutional Guide to DHEW Policy on Protection of Human Subjects. Washington, D.C. U.S. Government Printing Office, 1971.

"Protection of Human Subjects: Technical Amendments. 45 CFR 46." *Federal Register: Rules and Regulations* 40 (No. 50, March 13, 1975):11854–11858.

"Protection of Human Subjects: Proposed Policy," *Federal Register* 39 (August 23, 1974):30648–30657.

"Protection of Human Subjects: Fetuses, Pregnant Women, and In Vitro Fertilization," *Federal Register* 40 (August 8, 1975):33526–33552.

"Food and Drug Administration: Drugs for Human Use: Reorganization and Republication," *Federal Register* 39 (March 29, 1974):11684–11685, 11712–11718.

"Protection of Human Subjects: Proposed Policy," *Federal Register* 38 (October 9, 1973): Part II, pp. 27882–85.

"Protection of Human Subjects: Proposed Regulations on Research Involving Those Institutionalized as Mentally Disabled," *Federal Register* 43 (November 17, 1978):53950–56.

U.S. DEPARTMENT OF HEALTH AND HUMAN SERVICES (DHHS)

"Final Regulations Amending Basic HHS Policy for the Protection of Human Research Subjects: Final Rule: 45 CFR 46." *Federal Register: Rules and Regulations* 46 (No. 16, January 26, 1981):8366–8392.

"Additional Protections for Children Involved as Subjects in Research: Final Rule: 45 CFR 46." *Federal Register: Rules and Regulations* 48 (No. 46, March 8, 1983):9814–9820.

NATIONAL COMMISSION FOR THE PROTECTION OF HUMAN SUBJECTS OF BIOMEDICAL AND BEHAVIORAL RESEARCH

The Belmont Report: Ethical Principles and Guidelines for the Protection of Human Subjects of Research. Washington, D.C.: U.S. Government Printing Office, 1978.

Report and Recommendations: Research on the Fetus. Bethesda, MD: DHEW Publication No. (OS) 76-127, 1975.

Report and Recommendations: Research Involving Prisoners. Bethesda, MD: DHEW Publication No. (OS) 76-131, 1976.

Research Involving Children: Report and Recommendations. Washington, D.C.: U S Government Printing Office, 1977.

Report and Recommendations: Research Involving Those Institutionalized as Mentally Infirm. Bethesda, MD: DHEW Publication No. (OS) 78-0006, 1978.

Report and Recommendations: Institutional Review Boards. Bethesda, MD: DHEW Publication No. (OS) 78-0008, 1978.

U.S. SENATE SUBCOMMITTEE ON HEALTH OF THE COMMITTEE ON LABOR AND PUBLIC WELFARE

Quality of Health Care—Human Experimentation, 1973: Hearings Before the Subcommittee on Health of the Committee on Labor and Public Welfare United States

Senate, Ninety-Third Congress: First Session on S. 974, S. 878, S.J. Res. 71: Part 1.
Washington, D.C.: U.S. Government Printing Office, February 21 and 22, 1973.

Quality of Health Care—Human Experimentation, 1973. Hearings Before the Subcommittee on Health of the Committee on Labor and Public Welfare United States Senate, Ninety-Third Congress: First Session on S. 974, S. 878, S.J. Res. 71: Part 2.
Washington, D.C.: U.S. Government Printing Office, February 23 and March 6, 1973.

Quality of Health Care—Human Experimentation, 1973: Hearings Before the Subcommittee on Health of the Committee on Labor and Public Welfare United States Senate, Ninety-Third Congress: First Session on S. 974, S. 878, S.J. Res. 71: Part 3.
Washington, D.C.: U.S. Government Printing Office, March 7 and 8, 1973.

Quality of Health Care—Human Experimentation, 1973: Hearings Before the Subcommittee on Health of the Committee on Labor and Public Welfare United States Senate, Ninety-Third Congress: First Session on S. 974, S. 878, S.J. Res. 71: Part 4.
Washington, D.C.: U.S. Government Printing Office, April 30, June 28, 29, and July 10, 1973.

Federal Regulation of Human Experimentation (Washington, D.C.: U.S. Government Printing Office, 1975).

1. THE PATIENT AS PARTNER

1. H. K. Beecher, "Ethics and Clinical Research," *New England Journal of Medicine* 274 (1966):1354–60.

2. J. H. Jones, *Bad Blood* (New York: The Free Press, 1981).

3. R. M. Veatch, "Experimental Pregnancy: The Ethical Complexities of Experimentation with Oral Contraceptives," *Hastings Center Report* 1 (1971):2–3.

4. Jay Katz, ed., *Experimentation with Human Beings* (New York: Russell Sage Foundation, 1972), p. 9.

5. Blocker Heart Attack Trial Research Group, "A Randomized Trial of Propranolol in Patients with Acute Myocardial Infarction," *Journal of the American Medical Association* 247 (1982):1707–1714.

6. "What Are the Bounds of Decent Practice?" *Nature* 233 (1971):438–39.

7. R. M. Veatch, "Case Study: Risk-Taking in Cancer Chemotherapy," *IRB* 1 (August–September 1975):4–6.

8. DHHS, "Final Regulations."

9. A. M. Capron, "Informed Consent in Catastrophic Disease Research and Treatment," *University of Pennsylvania Law Review* 123 (1974):406; J. Katz, "Informed Consent—A Fairy Tale? Law's Vision," *University of Pittsburgh Law Review* 39 (1977):154–58; and L. L. Riskin, "Informed Consent: Looking for Action," *University of Illinois Law Forum* 39 (1975):580–611.

10. R. R. Faden, C. Lewis, C. Becker, A. I. Faden, and J. Freeman, "Disclosure Standards and Informed Consent," *Journal of Health and Political Policy Law* 6 (Summer 1981):255–84; and R. R. Faden, C. Becker, C. Lewis, J. Freeman, and A. I. Faden, "Disclosure of Information to Patients in Medical Care," *Medical Care* 19 (1981):718–33.

11. K. Lebacqz, "Justice and Human Research," *Justice and Health Care*, ed. E. E. Shelp (Dordrecht, Holland: D. Reidel, 1981), pp. 179–91; National Commission for the Protection of Human Subjects of Biomedical and Behavioral Research, *The Belmont Report*; DHHS, "Final Regulations."

12. Veatch, "Case Study."

2. DOING GOOD: BENEFICENCE AS THE MINIMAL JUSTIFICATION FOR RESEARCH

1. Claude Bernard, *An Introduction to the Study of Experimental Medicine*, tr. Henry Copley Greene, A.M. (New York: Dover Publications, Inc., 1957), p. 102.

2. Thomas Percival, *Percival's Medical Ethics* (1803; reprint ed. Chauncey D. Leake, Baltimore: Williams and Wilkins, 1927), p. 76.

3. Robert J. Levine, *Ethics and Regulation of Clinical Research* (Baltimore: Urban & Schwarzenberg, 1981), pp. 1–8.

4. World Medical Association (WMA), "Declaration of Geneva," *World Medical Journal* 3 (1956), supplement, pp. 10–12; reprinted in *Encyclopedia of Bioethics*, vol. 4, ed. Warren T. Reich (New York: The Free Press, 1978), p. 1749.

5. WMA, "International Code of Medical Ethics," in *Encyclopedia of Bioethics*, vol. 4, p. 1750.

6. WMA, "Declaration of Helsinki," in *Encyclopedia of Bioethics*, vol. 4, p. 1770.

7. Robert M. Veatch, *A Theory of Medical Ethics* (New York: Basic Books, 1981), pp. 160–61; Albert R. Jonsen, "Do No Harm: Axiom of Medical Ethics," in *Philosophical Medical Ethics: Its Nature and Significance*, ed. Stuart F. Spicker and H. Tristram Engelhardt, Jr. (Boston: D. Reidel Publishing Co., 1977), pp. 27–41.

8. Veatch, *A Theory of Medical Ethics*, pp. 159–64.

9. Jonsen, "Do No Harm," pp. 36–38.

10. W. D. Ross, *Foundations of Ethics* (Oxford: Oxford University Press, 1939), p. 75; William Frankena, *Ethics*, 2d ed. (Englewod Cliffs, New Jersey: Prentice-Hall, 1973), p. 47; Tom L. Beauchamp and James F. Childress, eds., *Principles of Biomedical Ethics*, 2d ed. (New York: Oxford University Press, 1983), p. 107.

11. James M. McCartney, "Encephalitis and Ara-A: An Ethical Case Study," *The Hastings Center Report* 8 (December 1978):7; Lawrence M. Friedman, "A Randomized Trial of Propranolol in Patients with Acute Myocardial Infarction," *Journal of the American Medical Association* 247 (March 26, 1982):1709–10.

12. Jay Katz, ed., *Experimentation with Human Beings* (New York: Russell Sage Foundation, 1972), p. 305.

13. *Ibid.*

14. John Rawls, "Two Concepts of Rules," *Philosophical Review* 44 (1955):3–32.

15. David Lyons, *Forms and Limits of Utilitarianism* (Oxford: Oxford University Press, 1965).

16. Rawls, "Two Concepts."

17. Beauchamp and Childress, *Principles of Biomedical Ethics;* National Commission for the Protection of Human Subjects, *The Belmont Report;* Veatch, *Theory of Medical Ethics.*

18. Veatch, *Theory of Medical Ethics*, pp. 177–287.

19. DHHS, "Final Regulations," p. 8389.

20. Veatch, *Theory of Medical Ethics*, pp. 295–305.

21. John Rawls, *A Theory of Justice* (Cambridge, Massachusetts: Harvard University Press, 1971), pp. 42–43.

22. DHHS, "Final Regulations," p. 8387.

23. DHEW, "Protection of Human Subjects."

24. *Ibid.*, p. 18917.

25. DHHS, "Final Regulations."

26. *Ibid.*, p. 8389.

3. THE PRINCIPLE OF AUTONOMY: THE FOUNDATION FOR INFORMED CONSENT

1. DHEW, "Protection of Human Subjects." See especially paragraph 46.2, p. 18917.

2. In fact I would stand with those who favor even more caution in getting consent for clinical care and so-called therapeutic experiments than non-therapeutic research because of the strong, sometimes coercive, interest a sick person has in maintaining the approval of medical professionals. See Robert J. Levine, "The Nature

and Definition of Informed Consent in Various Research Settings," in National Commission for the Protection of Human Subjects, *The Belmont Report*, Appendix vol. 1, pp. 3-1 to 3-91.

3. The alternative is to pack the requirements that consent be free and informed into the definition of consent. The Oxford English Dictionary has as its first definition "voluntary agreement to or acquiescence in what another proposes or desires; compliance, concurrence, permission." The ambiguity is apparently within the word itself. The first part of the definition includes the requirement of voluntariness while the latter synonyms do not. I prefer defining consent as the naked permission, leaving to the adjectives to specify that adequate consent must be free and informed. I believe that adds clarity and functionally leads reviewers to the proper questions to ask about a particular consent.

4. Hippocrates, *The Sacred Disease*, in W. H. S. Jones, ed., *Hippocrates* II, p. 134.

5. *Ibid.*

6. Ludwig Edelstein, "The Hippocratic Oath: Text, Translation, and Interpretation," in *Ancient Medicine* (Baltimore: Johns Hopkins University Press, 1976), pp. 3–63.

7. The oath states the patient-benefitting principle twice, first with regard to dietetic measures (one of the three elements of Pythagorean medicine): "I will apply dietetic measures for the benefit of the sick according to my ability and judgment." Later a more general form of the patient-benefit principle is repeated, this time without the explicit statement that the standard is to be the physician's own judgment, although this time the notion of intention is introduced: "Whatever houses I may visit, I will come for the benefit of the sick, remaining free of all intentional injustice. . . ." See text in Edelstein, *ibid.*, p. 6.

8. In addition to the fact that the patient-benefitting princple, if taken seriously, excludes all experimentation not done in the interests of the patient, it can also be criticized as being excessively individualistic (concentrating only on benefit to the individual, isolated patient) and paternalistic (using the physician's own judgment as the standard of reference). That it focuses exclusively on benefits and harms to the exclusion of other ethical questions such as rights and obligations inherent in action is a problem we shall discuss below.

9. It has been recognized that in special circumstances so-called non-therapeutic research might be undertaken on healthy subjects in the name of patient-benefit. If an individual were at high risk to a particular disease testing a vaccine on that person in the face of an epidemic might be justified on the grounds that the risk to the patient himself was less in conducting the trial of the vaccine than in letting the patient go unprotected. (See Paul Ramsey, *The Patient as Person* [New Haven: Yale University Press], pp. 15–16). Here, however, the principle of patient-benefit remains the norm. The judgment to include the patient in the test is made on strictly patient-benefitting grounds without consideration of benefit to others which might come from the knowledge gained.

10. See Robert J. Levine, "The Boundaries Between Biomedical or Behavioral Research and the Accepted and Routine Practice of Medicine," in *The Belmont Report*, Appendix, vol. 1, pp. 1–1 to 1–44.

11. Here I must explicitly reject the argument that some procedures undertaken where the two objectives of benefitting the patient and gaining knowledge both are present should not be seen as experimental. Bernard M. Dickens, for instance, argues that "If no orthodox treatment exists for the patient's condition (either because of the condition's novelty or because the orthodox treatment has become discredited by advances in medical knowledge) the physician's innovation will be nonexperimental" (Bernard M. Dickens, "What is a Medical Experiment?" *Canadian Medical Association Journal* 113 [October 4, 1974]:636.) That seems to me to simply be a

flagrant corruption of the term "experiment." It is one thing to say that under these circumstances there is no known better alternative; it is another to say that the trial of an unproved treatment is not experimental. Especially since he believes that a lower standard of consent may be required when a treatment is not experimental (a position which I reject in any case), much is at stake in the definitional debate. Certainly the patient ought to have the option of doing nothing in these circumstances, an option which by definition has not been shown to be any worse than the novel therapy.

12. "Food and Drug Administration: Consent for Use of Investigational New Drugs (IND) on Humans—Statement of Policy," text in Jay Katz, comp., *Experimentation with Human Beings* (New York: Russell Sage Foundation, 1972), p. 573. The same wording is reaffirmed in DHEW, "Food and Drug Administration: Drugs for Human Use," pp. 11684–685, 11712–718.

13. DHEW, *The Institutional Guide to DHEW Policy on Protection of Human Subjects* p. 8.

14. DHEW, "Protection of Human Subjects: Proposed Policy," 1973, pp. 27882–85.

15. DHEW, "Protection of Human Subjects," pp. 18914–920.

16. It has long been recognized that it may be reasonable to persist in requiring that a rule such as the informed-consent rule be followed even in individual cases where it appears that more good would come if the rule is violated. This is justified either on the grounds that the human being is sufficiently fallible that the rule is more likely to produce good on balance than individual judgment is or on the grounds that it is the nature of rules that they specify practices, practices which in turn might be chosen because they will produce more good than any other social practice. See John Rawls, "Two Concepts of Rules," *Philosophical Review* 64 (1955):3–32.

17. See Ralph J. Alfidi, "Informed Consent: A Study of Patient Reaction," *Journal of the American Medical Association* 216 (May 24, 1971):1325–29, for empirical evidence.

18. I recognize that the argument about consent in cases where the consent would do more harm than good implies that there may in fact be such cases. I am not prepared to concede that there are. If one recognizes that lack of consent per se may do harm—the patient may have unallayed fears, confusion about what behaviors are appropriate, etc.—then a case might be made that consent is always necessary on patient-benefitting grounds. For this discussion I presume, hypothetically, that consent might be contraindicated in some therapeutic experiment on patient-benefitting grounds.

In his important new discussion of the ethical foundations of experimentation Charles Fried develops the theme of "personal care" as the duty of the physician. (*Medical Experimentation: Personal Integrity and Social Policy* [New York: American Elsevier Publishing Co., Inc., 1974]). At one point he uses a qualified argument of "therapeutic privilege," that is, the argument that information could be withheld on grounds of patient benefit (p. 22). Later, however, when he develops the theme of "personal care," he makes the claim that personal care involves a notion of rights which belong to the patient which seem to be independent of consequences. These rights include "a right to know all relevant details" (p. 101), autonomy, trust, and "the right to be treated without deceit or violence" (p. 103). If, however, Fried perceives these to be rights inherent in personal care, it is hard to see how the physician has the "privilege" of overriding them when he believes (rightly or wrongly) that the overriding would be therapeutic. Therapeutic "privilege," if it exists at all, must be precisely that, a privilege the physician acquires because the patient has ceded the rights Fried has outlined.

19. World Medical Association, "Declaration of Helsinki," in *Encyclopedia of Bioethics*, vol. 4, ed. Warren T. Reich (New York: The Free Press, 1978), p. 1770.

20. American Medical Association Judicial Council, *Opinions and Reports of the*

Judicial Council (Chicago: A.M.A., 1971), pp. 11–12. Also see in addition to section 2, which commits the physician to improve medical knowledge, sections 1, 4, 9, and 10 where the physician is explicitly committed to serving society or other collective groups as well as the individual patient.

21. See Jeremy Bentham, *An Introduction to the Principles of Morals and Legislation;* John Stuart Mill, *Utilitarianism;* G. E. Moore, *Principia Ethica* (London: Cambridge University Press, 1903); and Henry Sidgwick, *The Methods of Ethics* (London: Macmillan and Co., Ltd., 1907).

22. William Harvey, *Exercitatio Anatomica de Motu Cordis et Sanguinis in Animalibus,* 1628. Also see Henry E. Sigerist, "William Harvey's Position in the History of European Thought," in *On the History of Medicine* (New York: MD Publications, 1960), pp. 184–92.

23. Chauncey D. Leake, ed., *Percival's Medical Ethics* (Huntington, New York: Robert E. Krieger Publishing Co., 1975), p. 76.

24. Claude Bernard, *An Introduction to the Study of Experimental Medicine* (New York: Dover, 1957), p. 102. Bernard certainly has gone further than even the classical utilitarians in claiming that experiments which may do good are obligatory. They would not be, according to the utilitarians, unless, all things considered, they would be likely to do more good than any other courses of action. Bernard, contrary to some interpretations of the negative formulation of the physician's duty *primum non nocere* (first, do no harm) seems to treat harms and benefits on the same scale.

25. This function corresponds to the point made by Katz and Capron that one purpose of informed consent is "to involve the public." Jay Katz and Alexander Morgan Capron, *Catastrophic Diseases: Who Decides What?* (New York: Russell Sage Foundation, 1975), p. 90; cf. Levine, "The Nature and Definition," p. 3–3.

26. DHEW, "Protection of Human Subjects," p. 18919.

27. DHHS, "Final Regulations."

28. *Ibid.,* p. 8390.

29. See Carl J. Wiggers, "Human Experimentation as Exemplified by the Career of Dr. William Beaumont," in *Clinical Investigations in Medicine: Legal, Ethical and Moral Aspects,* ed. Irving Ladimer and Roger W. Newman (Boston: Law-Medicine Research Institute, Boston University, 1963), pp. 119–25.

30. St. Martin bound himself to "serve, abide and continue with the said William Beaumont, wherever he shall go or travel or reside in any part of the world his *covenant servant* and diligently and faithfully . . . submit to assist and promote by all means in his power such philosophical or medical experiments as the said William shall direct or cause to be made on or in the stomach of him, the said Alexis, either through and by means of the aperture or opening thereto in the side of him, the said Alexis, or otherwise, and will obey, suffer and comply with all reasonable and proper orders of or experiments of the said William in relation thereto and in relation to the exhibiting and showing of his said stomach and the powers and properties thereto and of the appurtenances and the powers, properties and situation and state of the contents thereof." Text from William Beaumont, *Experiments and Observations on the Gastric Juice and the Physiology of Digestion,* 1833, cited in Henry Beecher, *Research and the Individual: Human Studies* (Boston: Little, Brown, 1970), p. 219.

31. See Michael R. LaChat, "Utilitarian Reasoning in Nazi Medical Policy: Some Preliminary Investigations," *Linacre Quarterly* 42 (Feb. 1975):14–37; for an important discussion of the general problems of utilitarian justification of human experimentation, see Ruth Macklin and Susan Sherwin, "Experimenting with Human Subjects: Philosophical Perspectives," *Case Western Reserve Law Review* 25 (1975):434–71.

32. "The experiment is to be such as to yield fruitful results for the good of

society, unprocurable by other methods or means of study." In Katz, *Experimentation*, p. 305.

33. Under this principle, it is further stated:

"This means that the person involved should have legal capacity to give consent; should be so situated as to be able to exercise free power of choice, without the intervention of any element of force, fraud, deceit, duress, over-reaching, or other ulterior form of constraint or coercion; and should have sufficient knowledge and comprehension of the elements of the subject matter involved as to enable him to make an understanding and enlightened decision. This latter element requires that before the acceptance of an affirmative decision by the experimental subject there should be made known to him the nature, duration, and purpose of the experiment; the method and means by which it is to be conducted; all inconveniences and hazards reasonably to be expected; and the effects upon his health or person which may possibly come from his participation in the experiment.

The duty and responsibility for ascertaining the quality of the consent rests upon each individual who initiates, directs, or engages in the experiment. It is a personal duty and responsibility which may not be delegated to another with impunity." In Katz, *Experimentation*, p. 305. Also see the interesting discussion in Bernard M. Dickens, "Contractual Aspects of Human Medical Experimentation," *University of Toronto Law Journal* 25 (1975):406–38.

34. *Carpenter* v. *Blake*, 60 Barb. 488 (N.Y. Sup. Ct. 1871).

35. *Jackson* v. *Burnham*, 20 Colo. 532, Pac. 577 (1895).

36. *Schloendorff* v. *New York Hospital*, 211 N.Y. 127, 129, 105 N.E. 92, 93 (1914), text in Katz, *Experimentation*, p. 526.

37. *Natanson* v. *Kline*, 186 Kan. 393, P. 2d 1093 (1960), text cited in Katz, *Experimentation*, p. 533.

38. *Fortner* v. *Koch*, 272 Mich. 272, N.W. 762 (1935).

39. DHEW, "Protection of Human Subjects," p. 18917.

40. DHHS, "Final Regulations," p. 8387.

41. I concede that someone with imagination might argue that there are indirect but serious risks—that mankind's respect for the genetically abnormal would change and that that, in turn, would have a psychological impact on the subject. If those risks are included, however, it seems that *any* research would have risks and that the proviso "if risk is involved" is meaningless.

It seems more plausible to say that the subject is not really at risk in the normal sense of the term, but that the rights and welfare of others are and that that is sufficient reason why some might want to refuse to consent to participate in the study.

42. I endorse Robert J. Levine's emphasis on explaining the "larger ultimate purpose" as well as the immediate one. See Levine, "The Nature and Definition," pp. 3-9 to 3-10.

43. See Immanuel Jakobovits, *Jewish Medical Ethics* (New York: Bloch Publishing Co., 1959), pp. 132–52; Fred Rosner, *Modern Medicine and Jewish Law* (New York: Yeshiva University Press, 1972), pp. 132–54; and David Bleich, "Medical Experimentation Upon Severed Organs," in his "Survey of Recent Halakhic Periodical Literature," *Tradition* 12 (Summer 1971):89–90.

44. See L. C. Epstein and L. Lasagna, "Obtaining Informed Consent: Form or Substance," *Archives of Internal Medicine* 123 (1969):682–88.

45. There are a number of variants on the professional standard: what is customary for physicians in the community to disclose, what physicians more generally in society or in a specialty group would disclose, or what the "reasonable physician" would disclose. All rely on a professional standard. See Leonard L. Riskin, "Informed Consent: Looking for the Action," *University of Illinois Law Forum* 39 (No. 4, 1975):580–611, especially 585–86.

46. *Natanson* v. *Kline*, 186 Kan. 393, P. 2d 1093 (1960), cited in Katz, *Experimentation*, p. 534.

47. California, Idaho, New York, Ohio, Oregon, Pennsylvania, Rhode Island, Washington, Wisconsin, and Tennessee, but cf. *Karp* v. *Cooley*, 349 F. Supp. 827 (S.D. Tex. 1972), affirmed 493 F. 2d 408 (5th Cir. 1974).

48. Riskin, "Informed Consent." Also see Don Harper Mills, "Whither Informed Consent?" *Journal of the American Medical Association* 229 (July 15, 1974):305–9, where Mills concludes (p. 305) that "the 'standard of practice' basis for judging the extent of disclosure will probably give way to a new rule of reasonableness; though what the courts believe to be reasonable disclosure may not necessarily be consistent with what physicians believe should be disclosed."

49. J. C. Garnham, "Some Observations on Informed Consent in Non-Therapeutic Research," *Journal of Medical Ethics* 1 (3 Sept. 1975):143–44. Many, including Garnham, still maintain that although informed consent of patient or subject is impossible, some consent should still be obtained. There seems to be an inconsistency in this position.

50. Of course, the same point can be made on patient- or subject-benefitting grounds if one holds that determining what is beneficial to the patient/subject is dependent upon the subject's own values. The fact that the researcher or the research community would find some piece of information irrelevant, given the researcher's values or the values of the research community as a whole, cannot be taken to imply that it would be irrelevant in another value context.

51. *Berkey* v. *Anderson*, 1 Cal. App. 3d 790, 805, 82 Cal. Rptr. 67, 78 (1969).

52. The implications of the reasonable-person court decisions for the composition of human experimentation committees and the questions they must answer is explored in greater detail in Robert M. Veatch, "Human Experimental Committees: Professional or Representative?" *Hastings Center Report* 5 (October 1975):31–40.

53. Norman Fost, "A Surrogate System for Informed Consent," *Journal of the American Medical Association* 233 (Aug. 18, 1975):800–803.

54. This interpretation differs slightly from that of Robert J. Levine, "The Nature and Definition," p. 3–19. He says that the reasonable-person standard "puts the particular physician or investigator in the precarious position of having to know in advance what harms a particular patient or subject might consider material after they occur." I agree that the physician is placed in a precarious position, but I do not think it is quite that precarious. My reading of the case law is that the physician must simply disclose what the reasonable person would find meaningful or useful. This should be modified when the physician has reason to believe that the individual patient or subject differs from that reasonable-person view, but, unless the physician has negligently or maliciously avoided the discovery that the individual patient differs from the reasonable person, I do not see that he would be held to the standard of that (deviant) patient or subject. Of course, the physician is still in a precarious position because this series of cases makes clear that the physician's own judgment or even the consensus of medical professionals cannot be taken to adequately predict what the reasonable person would want to know. This does mean, however, that an all-lay committee made up of individuals reasonably presumed to be reasonable would be a plausible test of the adequacy of the information, unless there were information to the contrary about the individual subject. Levine goes on (p. 3-20) to introduce the reasonable-person standard, but without qualifying it for the case when the researcher knows or should know that the subject differs from that reasonable person.

55. DHHS, "Final Regulations."

56. For a fuller discussion of these elements see the author's "Ethical Principles of Medical Experimentation," in *Ethical and Legal Issues of Social Experimentation*, ed. Alice M. Rivlin and P. Michael Timpane (Washington: The Brookings Institution, 1975), pp. 21–59, especially pp. 52–57.

57. See a fuller discussion of this issue below.

58. The specific mention of "inconveniences" occurs in the Nuremberg Code. Its omission has been taken as justifying non-disclosure of inconveniences by some review committee members although "inconveniences" could be taken to be subsumed in "risks." That "discomforts" is listed as separate from "risks" can be cited to support the claim that "inconveniences" are not to be taken as risks.

59. DHHS, "Final Regulations."

60. Robert J. Levine, "The Nature and Definition," pp. 3-10, 3-11, 3-25.

61. Ibid., p. 3-57. Cf. DHEW, "Protection of Human Subjects," p. 18919.

62. See Louis Lasagna, The Conflict of Interest Between Physician as Therapist and as Experimenter (Philadelphia: Society for Health and Human Values, 1975).

63. John Stuart Mill, On Liberty (New York: Liberal Arts Press, 1956), p. 114, where he argues that "for such actions as are prejudicial to the interests of others, the individual is accountable and may be subjected either to social or to legal punishment if society is of opinion that the one or the other is requisite for its protection."

64. Ibid., p. 125.

65. This is the term preferred by Alexander Morgan Capron, "Legal Considerations Affecting Clinical Pharmacological Studies in Children," Clinical Research 21 (1972):141–50.

66. Paul Ramsey, The Patient as Person, Chapter 1.

67. The argument here is related to Richard McCormick's in "Proxy Consent in the Experimentation Situation," Perspectives in Biology and Medicine 18 (Autumn 1974):2–20.

68. G. Emmett Raitt, "The Minor's Right to Consent to Medical Treatment: A Corollary of the Constitutional Right of Privacy," Southern California Law Review 48 (1975):1417–56.

69. In re the matter of Karen Quinlan: an alleged incompetent: Superior Court of New Jersey, Chancery Division, Morris County, Docket No. C-201-75; Winters v. Miller, 446 F. 2d 65 (C.A.2, May 26, 1971).

70. New York City Health and Hospitals Corporation and Edward A. Stolzenberg, Associate Director, Bellevue Hospital, Petitioners, v. Paula Stein, a patient, respondent, 335 N.Y. 2d 461.

71. In re appointment of a guardian of the person of Maida Yetter, Docket No. 1973-533 (Pa. Ct. of Common Pleas, Northampton Co. Orphan's Ct., June 6, 1973).

72. N.Y. State Mental Hygiene Law, Article 15, "Rights of Patients," Section 15.03, Point (b)4.

73. I have heard this suggested in personal communication with Karen Lebacqz and, independently, by Roy Branson. Whether the system would work, I do not know. Possibly prison officials or dominant prisoners would gain control of the funds in some cases leading to their inequitable use. Also it is not clear why drug companies and others wanting to do research would choose prisoners as subjects under these conditions. In order to get subjects in a controlled environment for long periods of time, they might recruit students who would agree to spend weeks in a controlled institution in exchange for offerings of summer school courses, room and board at the researcher's expense. Whether an offer to an economically deprived group such as students would be seen as less coercive than an offer to prisoners, I do not know, but at least institutional review and control might be more dependable and the danger of use of research for retribution would be eliminated.

74. American Medical Association of Delegates, "Resolution on Disapproval of Participation in Scientific Experiments by Inmates of Penal Institutions," text in Henry Beecher, Research and the Individual, p. 225. This position may also be rooted in the concern for protecting the public interest insofar as research participation leads to earlier release from prison. It would not directly justify opposition to meritorious or commendatory citation, however.

75. We have already argued that the positions of private groups of professionals should not be persuasive in setting public policy. They are often committed to special value stances not shared by the general public. Thus the acceptance by the American Psychological Association of deception and even lying—presumably on the justification of the social benefits to be obtained—should not be terribly relevant to the Commission. The Association's unique commitment to the social value of the particular type of knowledge gained should not influence commissioners who have a public obligation to protect constitutionally guaranteed rights. See American Psychological Association, *Ethical Principles in the Conduct of Research With Human Participants* (Washington, D.C.: A.P.A., 1973), pp. 29–35; cf. Code of Ethics, American Sociological Association, which says obliquely, "Just as sociologists must not distort or manipulate truth to serve untruthful ends, so too they must not manipulate persons to serve their quest for truth."

76. Hans Jonas, *Philosophical Essays* (Englewood Cliffs, N.J.: Prentice-Hall, 1974), p. 126.

77. See the qualifications of this statement related to a possible theory of justice below.

78. I believe this is a more explicit principle and more precise requirement than Levine advocates. See Levine, "The Nature and Definition," p. 3–30.

79. DHEW, "Protection of Human Subjects: Proposed Policy," 1974, pp. 30653–654.

80. DHEW, "Protection of Human Subjects: Fetuses, Pregnant Women, and In Vitro Fertilization," pp. 33526–52. I also support third-party scrutiny proposals as set forth by Levine, "The Nature and Definition," pp. 3–46 to 3–52. However, I feel such third parties should be used only with the consent of the subject. Discussing the proposed research first with the next of kin and/or a physician not connected with the research is certainly a violation of the individual's right to confidentiality. It should be clear, however, that third parties must be independent of the researcher and his or her staff. Thus the debate between Don Harper Mills and Alan Meisel over whether the physician or nurses and physician assistants associated with them would be better witnesses of the consent may be misplaced. While certainly the physician or researcher cannot be an adequate witness of a consent contract between himself and the patient or subject, those working under his supervision would not be adequate either. See Alan Meisel, "Informed Consent—The Rebuttal," *Journal of the American Medical Association* 234 (Nov. 10, 1975):615; and Don Harper Mills, "Informed Consent—The Rejoinder," *Journal of the American Medical Association* 234 (Nov. 10, 1975):616.

81. "Position Statement of the American Federation for Clinical Research on the DHEW Proposed Rules on Protection of Human Subjects," *Clinical Research* 23 (1975):53–60.

82. John Rawls, *A Theory of Justice* (Cambridge, Mass.: Harvard University Press, 1971).

83. See Brian Barry, *The Liberal Theory of Justice* (New York: Oxford University Press, 1973); and Robert M. Veatch, "What Is a Just Health Care Delivery?" in *Ethics and Health Policy*, ed. Robert M. Veatch and Roy Branson (Cambridge, Mass.: Ballinger Press, forthcoming).

84. See Macklin and Sherwin, "Experimenting with Human Subjects."

4. JUSTICE AND RESEARCH DESIGN

1. K. Lebacqz, "Justice and Human Research," in *Justice and Health Care*, ed. E. E. Shelp (Dordrecht, Holland: D. Reidel Publishing Co., 1981), pp. 179–91.

2. Robert J. Levine, *Ethics and Regulation of Clinical Research* (Baltimore: Urban & Schwarzenberg, 1981), pp. 61–66, 129–31.

3. C. Fried, *Medical Experimentation: Personal Integrity and Social Policy.* (New York: American Elsevier, 1974).

4. National Commission for the Protection of Human Subjects, *The Belmont Report*, pp. 4–10.

5. DHEW, "Protection of Human Subjects: Proposed Regulations on Research Involving Those Institutionalized as Mentally Disabled," pp. 53955-56.

6. DHHS, "Final Regulations," p. 8389.

7. Aristotle, *Nicomachean Ethics*, tr. Martin Ostwald (Indianapolis: Bobbs-Merrill, 1962), 111–15.

8. *Ibid.*, pp. 115–20.

9. R. Nozick, *Anarchy, State and Utopia* (New York: Basic Books, Inc., 1974).

10. J. S. Mill, *Utilitarianism* (1863; reprint ed. Samuel Gorovitz, Indianapolis: Bobbs-Merrill Co., Inc., 1971), pp. 42–57.

11. J. Rawls, *A Theory of Justice* (Cambridge: Harvard University Press, 1971).

12. Robert J. Levine and Karen A. Lebacqz, "Ethical Considerations in Clinical Trials," *Clinical Pharmacology and Therapeutics* 25 (1979):728–41.

13. Levine, *Ethics*, pp. 64–66.

14. B. Barry, *The Liberal Theory of Justice: A Critical Examination of the Principal Doctrines in A Theory of Justice by John Rawls* (Oxford: Clarendon Press, 1973).

15. R. Veatch, *A Theory of Medical Ethics* (New York: Basic Books, Inc., 1981), p. 265.

16. C. Ake, "Justice as Equality," *Philosophy and Public Affairs* 5 (1975):71.

17. *The Belmont Report*, p. 2.

18. DHHS, "Final Regulations," p. 8366.

19. W. D. Ross, *The Right and The Good* (Oxford: Oxford University Press, 1930), p. 19.

20. Veatch, *Theory of Medical Ethics*, pp. 303–5.

21. R. Veatch, "Three Theories of Informed Consent: The Philosophical Foundations and Policy Implications," in *The Belmont Report*, pp. 26–48.

22. A. M. Rivlin and P. M. Timpane, eds., *Ethical and Legal Issues of Social Experimentation* (Washington, D.C.: The Brookings Institution, 1975), pp. 1–4.

23. *Ibid.*, p. 4.

5. FEDERAL REGULATION OF MEDICINE AND BIOMEDICAL RESEARCH: POWER, AUTHORITY, AND LEGITIMACY

1. Talcott Parsons, *The Social System* (New York: Free Press, 1951), pp. 36–58.

2. Max Weber, *The Theory of Social and Economic Organization* (New York: Free Press, 1964), pp. 324–86.

3. L. Lasagna, "Drug Discovery and Introduction: Regulation and Overregulation," *Clinical Pharmacology and Therapeutics* 20(5):507–11.

4. Kurt Baier, *The Moral Point of View* (New York: Random House, 1965), pp. 90–92.

5. Peter Berger, *The Sacred Canopy* (Garden City, New York: Doubleday, 1967), pp. 179–88.

6. Chester Swinyard, *Decision Making and the Defective Newborn* (Springfield, Ill.: Charles C. Thomas, 1978), pp. 183–90; Angela R. Holder, "Liability and the IRB Member: The Legal Aspects," *IRB: A Review of Human Subjects Research* 1 (No. 3, May 1979):135–57.

7. John Stuart Mill, *On Liberty* (New York: The Liberal Arts Press, 1956).

8. Robert M. Veatch, "Professional Medical Ethics: The Grounding of Its Principles," *Journal of Medicine and Philosophy* 4 (March 1979):1–19.

9. Robert M. Veatch, *Value-Freedom in Science and Technology* (Missoula, Montana: Scholars Press, 1976).

10. Edmund C. Pellegrino, "Toward an Expanded Medical Ethics: The Hippocratic Ethic Revisited," in *Hippocrates Revisited: A Search for Meaning*, ed. Roger J. Bulger (New York: Medcom Press, 1973), pp. 133–47.

11. Richard Magraw, "Science and Humanism: Medicine and Existential Anguish," in *Hippocrates Revisited*, pp. 148–57.

12. William F. May, "Code, Covenant, Contract, or Philanthropy?" *Hastings Center Report* 5 (December 1975):29–38.

13. Joel Feinberg, *Doing and Deserving: Essays in the Theory of Responsibility* (Princeton, N.J.: Princeton University Press, 1970), pp. 5–9.

14. Darrel W. Amundsen, "The Physician's Obligation to Prolong Life: A Medical Duty without Classical Roots," *Hastings Center Report* 8 (August 1978):28.

15. Robert M. Veatch, *Death, Dying, and the Biological Revolution* (New Haven, Conn.: Yale University Press, 1976), pp. 21–76.

16. William C. Charron, "Death: A Philosophical Perspective on the Legal Definitions," *Washington University Law Quarterly* 4 (1975):979–1008.

17. Hans Jonas, "Against the Stream: Comments on the Definition and Redefinition of Death," in *Philosophical Essays: From Ancient Creed to Technological Man* (Englewood Cliffs, N.J.: Prentice-Hall, Inc., 1974), pp. 132–40.

18. J. B. Brierley, J. A. H. Adam, D. I. Graham, and J. A. Simpson, "Neocortical Death after Cardiac Arrest," *Lancet*, September 11, 1971, pp. 560–65; Veatch, *Death, Dying, and the Biological Revolution*, pp. 13–30.

19. Bernard Barber, "Some Problems in the Sociology of the Professions," *Daedalus* 92 (1963):669–88.

20. May, "Code, Covenant, Contract, or Philanthropy?" pp. 29–31.

21. Bernard Barber et al., *Research on Human Subjects* (New York: Russell Sage, 1973), p. 51.

6. FEDERAL REGULATIONS: PROGRESS AND PROBLEMS

1. DHHS, "Final Regulations," pp. 8366–92.

2. *Ibid.*, p. 8389.

3. *Ibid.*

4. *Ibid.*, p. 8390.

5. William Curran, "Governmental Regulation of the Use of Human Subjects in Medical Research: The Approach to Two Federal Agencies," *Daedalus* 98 (Spring 1969):542–49; Mark Frankel, "The Development of Policy Guidelines Governing Human Experimentation in the United States: A Case Study of Public Policy Making for Science and Technology," *Ethics in Science and Medicine* 2 (May 1975):43–59.

6. "Statement of Robert Veatch, Ph.D., Hastings Institute, Hastings-on-Hudson, N.Y.," in U.S. Senate Subcommittee on Health, *Quality of Health Care—Human Experimentation, 1973* (hereafter *Hearings*), Part 1, pp. 265–75.

7. *Hearings*, Part 1; Part 2; Part 3; and Part 4.

8. National Commission for the Protection of Human Subjects of Biomedical and Behavioral Research (hereafter Commission). *Report and Recommendations: Research on the Fetus.*

9. Commission, *Report and Recommendations: Research Involving Prisoners.*

10. Commission, *Research Involving Children: Report and Recommendations.*

11. Commission, *Report and Recommendations: Research Involving Those Institutionalized as Mentally Infirm.*

12. Commission, *Report and Recommendations: Institutional Review Boards.*

13. Commission, *The Belmont Report.*

14. John Rawls, *A Theory of Justice* (Cambridge, Massachusetts: Harvard University Press, 1971).

15. Laws of New York 1975, "Article 24-A: Protection of Human Subjects," *Public Health—Human Research—Protection of Subjects: Chapter 450*, pp. 646–49.

16. Commission, *Report and Recommendations: Institutional Review Boards*.

17. DHHS, "Final Regulations," p. 8387.

18. *Ibid.*, p. 8392.

19. *Ibid.*, p. 8389.

20. *Ibid.*, p. 8390.

21. *Ibid.*

22. Commission, *Report and Recommendations: Institutional Review Boards*, pp. 26–27.

23. DHHS, "Final Regulations," p. 8390.

24. *Ibid.*

25. *Ibid.*, p. 8387.

26. Commission, *Report and Recommendations: Institutional Review Boards*, p. 36.

7. INSTITUTIONAL REVIEW BOARDS: PROFESSIONAL OR REPRESENTATIVE?

1. Thomas Percival, *Percival's Medical Ethics* (1803; reprint ed., Chauncey D. Leake, Baltimore: Williams and Wilkins, 1927), p. 76.

2. Mark Frankel, "The Development of Policy Guidelines Governing Human Experimentation in the United States: A Case Study of Public Policy Making for Science and Technology," *Ethics in Science and Medicine*, (May 1975):43–59; also see U.S. Senate Subcommittee on Health, *Federal Regulation of Human Experimentation*.

3. *Ibid.*, p. 13.

4. William Curran, "Governmental Regulation of the Use of Human Subjects in Medical Research: The Approach of Two Federal Agencies," *Daedalus* (Spring 1969):547.

5. *Ibid.*, p. 549.

6. Robert B. Livingston, "Progress Report on Survey of Moral and Ethical Aspects of Clinical Investigation," November 1964, memo to Director, NIH.

7. James A. Shannon, "Moral and Ethical Aspects of Clinical Investigation," letter of transmittal to the U.S. Surgeon General.

8. Public Health Service, "Requirements for Review to Insure the Rights and Welfare of Individuals," in Henry Beecher, *Research and the Individual: Human Studies* (Boston: Little, Brown, 1970), pp. 293–96.

9. Jay Katz, ed., *Experimentation with Human Beings* (New York: Russell Sage, 1972), pp. 886–89.

10. DHHS, "Final Regulations," pp. 8387–88.

11. DHEW, "Protection of Human Subjects," p. 18918.

12. DHEW, *The Institutional Guide to DHEW Policy on Protection of Human Subjects*, p. 4.

13. DHEW, "Protection of Human Subjects," p. 18918.

14. DHHS, "Final Regulations," p. 8388.

15. DHEW, *The Institutional Guide*, p. 4.

16. DHEW, "Protection of Human Subjects," p. 18918.

17. *Ibid.*

18. National Commission for the Protection of Human Subjects of Biomedical and Behavioral Research (hereafter Commission), *Report and Recommendations: Institutional Review Boards*, p. 14.

19. DHHS, "Final Regulations," p. 8388.

20. Commission, *Report and Recommendations: Institutional Review Boards,* p. 13.

21. *Ibid.,* p. 15.

22. DHHS, "Final Regulations," p. 8388.

23. Bernard Barber et al., *Research on Human Subjects: Problems of Social Control in Medical Experimentation* (New York: Russell Sage, 1973), p. 152; Bradford H. Gray, *Human Subjects in Medical Experimentation* (New York: Wiley-Interscience, 1975).

24. Barber et al., *Research on Human Subjects,* p. 153.

25. David S. Rubsamen, "Changes in Informed Consent," *Medical World News,* February 9, 1973, pp. 66–67; Joseph E. Simonaitis, "Recent Decisions on Informed Consent," *Journal of the American Medical Association* 221 (July 24, 1972):441–42; Joseph E. Simonaitis, "More About Informed Consent: Part I," *Journal of the American Medical Association* 224 (June 25, 1973):1831–32.

26. J. A. F. Stoner, "A Comparison of Individual and Group Decisions Involving Risk" (Master's thesis, School of Industrial Management, Massachusetts Institute of Technology, 1961).

27. Colin Fraser et al., "Risky Shifts, Cautious Shifts and Group Polarization," *European Journal of Social Psychology* 1 (1971):7–30.

28. DHHS, "Final Regulations," p. 8388.

8. LIABILITY AND THE IRB MEMBER: THE ETHICAL ASPECTS

1. Angela R. Holder, "Liability and the IRB Member: The Legal Aspects," *IRB: A Review of Human Subjects Research* 1 (No. 3, May 1979):7–8.

2. National Commission for the Protection of Human Subjects (hereafter Commission), *The Belmont Report,* p. 11.

3. Angela R. Holder, "Liability and the IRB Member," p. 8.

4. Commission, *Report and Recommendations: Institutional Review Boards,* p. 82.

5. DHHS, "Final Regulations," p. 8389.

6. Commission, *Institutional Review Boards,* pp. 82–86.

9. JUSTICE AND THE SEMI-RANDOMIZED CLINICAL TRIAL

1. E. J. Freireich and E. A. Gehan, "The Limitations of the Randomized Clinical Trial," *Methods in Cancer Research* 17:277–309.

2. E. J. Freireich, "Informed Consent versus Pre-randomization," in *Adjuvant Therapy of Cancer III,* ed. S. E. Salmon and S. E. Jones (New York: Grune & Stratton, Inc., 1981), pp. 53–62.

3. H. O. Conn, "Therapeutic Portacaval Anastomosis: To Shunt or Not to Shunt," *Gastroenterology* (1974):1067.

4. *Ibid.,* p. 1070.

10. SUBJECTS WHO BENEFIT BECAUSE THEY ARE MISERABLE

1. Thomas Percival, *Percival's Medical Ethics* (1803; reprint ed. Chauncey D. Leake, Baltimore: Williams and Wilkins, 1927), p. 76.

2. S. Krugman, R. Ward, J. P. Giles, O. Bodansky, and A. M. Jacobs, "Infectious Hepatitis: Detection of Virus during the Incubation Period and in Clinically Inapparent Infection," *New England Journal of Medicine* 261 (1959):729–34.

3. Presentation by Dr. Ellen Isaacs, Proceedings of The Symposium on Ethical Issues in Human Experimentation: The Case Willowbrook State Hospital Research, May 4, 1972, sponsored by The Student Council of New York University School of Medicine, Published by the Urban Health Affairs Program New York University Medical Center, 1972 (hereafter Willowbrook Symposium), p. 20; Henry K. Beecher, *Research and the Individual: Human Studies* (Boston: Little, Brown and Company, 1970), pp. 122–27; Henry K. Beecher, "Ethics and Clinical Research," *New England Journal of Medicine* 274 (1966):1354–60.

4. See for example the letters by Stephen Goldby (*The Lancet*, April 10, 1971); by Saul Krugman and Samuel Shapiro (*The Lancet*, May 8, 1971); by Edward N. Willey (*The Lancet*, May 22, 1971); by Joan Pott Giles (*The Lancet*, May 29, 1971); by M. H. Pappworth (*The Lancet*, June 5, 1971); and by Geoffrey Edsall (*The Lancet*, July 10, 1971).

5. "International Code of Medical Ethics," The General Assembly of the World Medical Association, London, England, 1949, in Beecher, *Research and the Individual: Human Studies*, p. 236.

6. "Principles for Those in Research and Experimentation," The General Assembly of the World Medical Association, 1954, in Beecher, *Research and the Individual: Human Studies*, p. 240.

7. "Declaration of Helsinki," World Medical Association, 1964, in Beecher, *Research and the Individual: Human Studies*, p. 277.

8. Saul Krugman, "Experiments at the Willowbrook State School," A Letter to the Editor, *The Lancet*, May 8, 1971, pp. 966–67.

9. Presentation by Dr. Saul Krugman, Willowbrook Symposium, p. 6.

10. Saul Krugman, "Experiments," p. 966.

11. Isaacs, p. 20.

12. DHHS, "Additional Protections for Children Involved as Subjects in Research," p. 9819.

13. Ernst Troeltsch, "Das stoische-christliche Naturrecht und die moderne profane Naturrecht," in *Gesammelte Schriften, IV* (Tubingen: Verlag J. C. B. Mohr [Paul Siebeck], 1925), pp. 166–91.

11. THE PROBLEM OF PRELIMINARY DATA: LONGITUDINAL STUDIES, SEQUENTIAL DESIGN, AND GRANT RENEWALS

1. For a summary of the history and methods of sequential design, see: P. Armitragem, *Sequential Medical Trials*, 2d ed. (New York: Halsted Press [distributed by John Wiley & Sons, Inc.], 1975).

2. P. C. Elwood et al., "A Randomized Controlled Trial of Acetylsalicylic Acid in the Secondary Prevention of Mortality from Myocardial Infarction," *British Medical Journal* 1 (March 9, 1974):436–40.

3. DHHS, "Final Regulations," p. 8389.

12. INFORMED CONSENT: THE USE OF LAY SURROGATES TO DETERMINE HOW MUCH INFORMATION SHOULD BE TRANSMITTED

1. R. J. Alfidi, "Informed Consent: A Study of Patient Reaction," *Journal of the American Medical Association* 216 (1971):1325–29.

2. R. J. Alfidi, "Informed Consent and Special Procedure," *Cleveland Clinic Quarterly* 40 (1973):21–25.

3. R. J. Alfidi, "Controversy, Alternatives, and Decisions in Complying with the Legal Doctrine of Informed Consent," *Radiology* 114 (1975):231–34.

4. G. Robinson and A. Merav, "Informed Consent: Recall by Patients Tested Postoperatively," *Annals of Thoracic Surgery* 22 (1976):209–12.

5. *Natanson v. Kline,* 187 Kan. 186, 350 P. 2d 1093 (1960).

6. *Berkey v. Anderson,* 1 Cal. App. 3d 790, 805, 82 Cal. Rptr. 67, 78 (1969).

7. *Cobbs v. Grant,* 8 Cal. 3d 229, 502 P. 2d 1, 104 Cal. Rptr. 505 (1972).

8. *Wilkinson v. Vesey,* 110 R.I. 606, 295 A. 2d 676 (1972).

9. *Canterbury v. Spence,* 464 F. 2d 772 (D.C. Cir.), cert. denied 409 U.S. 1064.

10. R. M. Veatch, "Three Theories of Informed Consent: Philosophical Foundations and Policy Implications," *The Belmont Report,* pp. 26–1 through 26–66.

11. R. M. Veatch, "Human Experimentation Committees: Professional or Representative?" *Hastings Center Report* 5 (1975):31–40.

12. N. C. Fost, "A Surrogate System for Informed Consent," *Journal of the American Medical Association* 223 (1975):800–803.

13. Reports and Recommendations of the National Immunization Work Groups, March 15, 1977. Submitted to the Office of the Assistant Secretary for Health: National Immunization Work Group on Consent.

14. DHHS, "Final Regulations," p. 8390.

13. LIMITS ON THE RIGHT TO PRIVACY: THE ETHICS OF RECORD SEARCHES AND OTHER USES OF PRIVATE MATERIALS

1. It is possible, however, for one to be a consequentialist and still hold that privacy may not be overridden by other considerations such as public safety, if one is a rule utilitarian who believes that taking this view will lead to the best consequences. Note, however, that this view does not in principle forbid invasions of privacy. If invasions of privacy are forbidden, it is not due to something inherently valuable about privacy itself. It is only because it just so happens that this will lead to the best possible consequences. Thus whether or not privacy rights should be overridden is entirely an empirical matter for the rule utilitarian. A rule utilitarian must admit that he or she would be forced to change positions if the empirical evidence were in opposition to his or her view.

2. DHHS, "Final Regulations," p. 8387.

3. E. L. Pattullo, "The Limits of the 'Right' of Privacy," *IRB: A Review of Human Subjects Research* 4 (April 1982):4.

4. DHHS, "Final Regulations," p. 8390.

5. See chapter 12 of this volume.

6. DHHS, "Final Regulations," p. 8387.

14. "EXPERIMENTAL" PREGNANCY: THE ETHICAL COMPLEXITIES OF EXPERIMENTATION WITH ORAL CONTRACEPTIVES

1. Henry K. Beecher, "Ethics and Clinical Research," *New England Journal of Medicine* 274 (1966):1353–60.

2. Joseph W. Goldzieher, Louis E. Moses, Eugene Averkin, Cora Scheel, and Ben Z. Taber, "A Placebo-Controlled Double-Blind Crossover Investigation of the Side Effects Attributed to Oral Contraceptives," *Fertility and Sterility* 22 (No. 9, September 1971):609–23.

3. *Ibid.,* p. 610.

4. "Placebo Stirs Pill 'Side Effects'," *Medical World News,* April 16, 1971, pp. 18–19.

5. *Ibid.,* p. 19.

6. *Ibid.*

7. *Ibid.*
8. *Ibid.*
9. *Ibid.*
10. *Ibid.*
11. *Ibid.*, p. 18.

15. CONTRACEPTION RESEARCH ON TEENAGERS: BEYOND CONSENT TO TREATMENT

1. National Commission for the Protection of Human Subjects of Biomedical and Behavioral Research (hereafter Commission), *Research Involving Children: Report and Recommendations* (Washington: GPO, 1977), pp. 85–87.
2. *Ibid.*, p. 18.
3. *Ibid.*, pp. 17–19.
4. DHHS, "Final Regulations," pp. 8389–90.
5. *Ibid.*, p. 8390.
6. Commission, *Research Involving Children*, pp. 5–6.
7. *Ibid.*, p. 4.
8. DHHS, "Additional Protections for Children Involved as Subjects in Research," p. 9820.

16. RESEARCH ON THE BRAIN-DEAD: A SPECIAL CASE OF RESEARCH ON "NON-CONSENTABLES"

1. Ronald A. Carson, Jaime L. Frias, and Richard J. Melker, "Case Study: Research with Brain-Dead Children," *IRB: A Review of Human Subjects Research* 3 (No. 1, January 1981):5.
2. *Ibid.*
3. *Ibid.*
4. National Commission for the Protection of Human Subjects of Biomedical and Behavioral Research, *Research Involving Children: Report and Recommendations*, p. 5.
5. DHHS, "Additional Protections for Children Involved as Subjects in Research," pp. 9814–20.
6. Robert M. Veatch, "Limits of Guardian Treatment Refusal: A Reasonableness Standard," *American Journal of Law and Medicine* 9(4, Winter 1984):427–68.
7. Carson, Frias, and Melker, "Case Study," p. 5.
8. *Ibid.*, p. 6.

17. RISK-TAKING IN CANCER CHEMOTHERAPY

1. DHHS, "Final Regulations," p. 8389.
2. *Ibid.*, p. 8366–92.
3. World Medical Association (WMA), "Declaration of Helsinki," in *Encyclopedia of Bioethics*, vol. 4, ed. Warren T. Reich (New York: The Free Press, 1978), pp. 1769–71.
4. "Nuremburg Code, 1946," in *Encyclopedia of Bioethics*, pp. 1764–65.
5. DHHS, "Final Regulations," p. 8366–92.
6. WMA, "Declaration of Helsinki," p. 1773.
7. *Natanson v. Kline* 186 Kan. 393, 350 P. 2d 1093 (1960), p. 533, in *Experimentation with Human Beings*, ed. Jay Katz (New York: Russell Sage Foundation, 1972).

18. THE ETHICS OF RESEARCH INVOLVING RADIATION

1. DHEW, "Protection of Human Subjects: Technical Amendments," p. 11854.

2. DHHS, "Final Regulations," p. 8366–92.

3. National Council on Radiation Protection and Measurements, "Basic Radiation Protection Criteria," NCRP Report No. 39 (Washington, 1980).

4. "The Totally Implantable Artificial Heart," Report by Artificial Heart Assessment Panel, National Heart and Lung Institute, June 1973, reprinted September 1973 (available from National Heart and Lung Institute, National Institutes of Health, Bethesda, MD 20014).

5. Richard McCormick, "Proxy Consent in the Experimentation Situation," in *How Brave a New World: Dilemmas in Bioethics* (Garden City, New York: Doubleday and Company, 1981), pp. 3–17.

6. *The Belmont Report*, p. 11.

7. Naomi Alazraki, "Evaluating Risk from Radiation for Research Subjects," *IRB: A Review of Human Subjects Research* 4 (No. 1, January 1982):3.

INDEX